© Copyright 2016 by Juniper Bowers. All rights reserved.

No part of this publication may be reproduced, stored in any retrieval system, or transmitted, in any form or by any means, electronic, mechanical, photo-copying, recording, or otherwise without the prior permission of the publisher, except for the quotation of brief passages in reviews.

Published by Juniper Bowers

San Lorenzo, NM

CIP data block info:`

TABLE OF CONTENTS

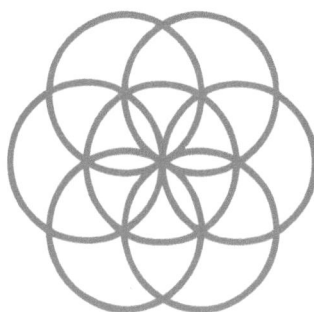

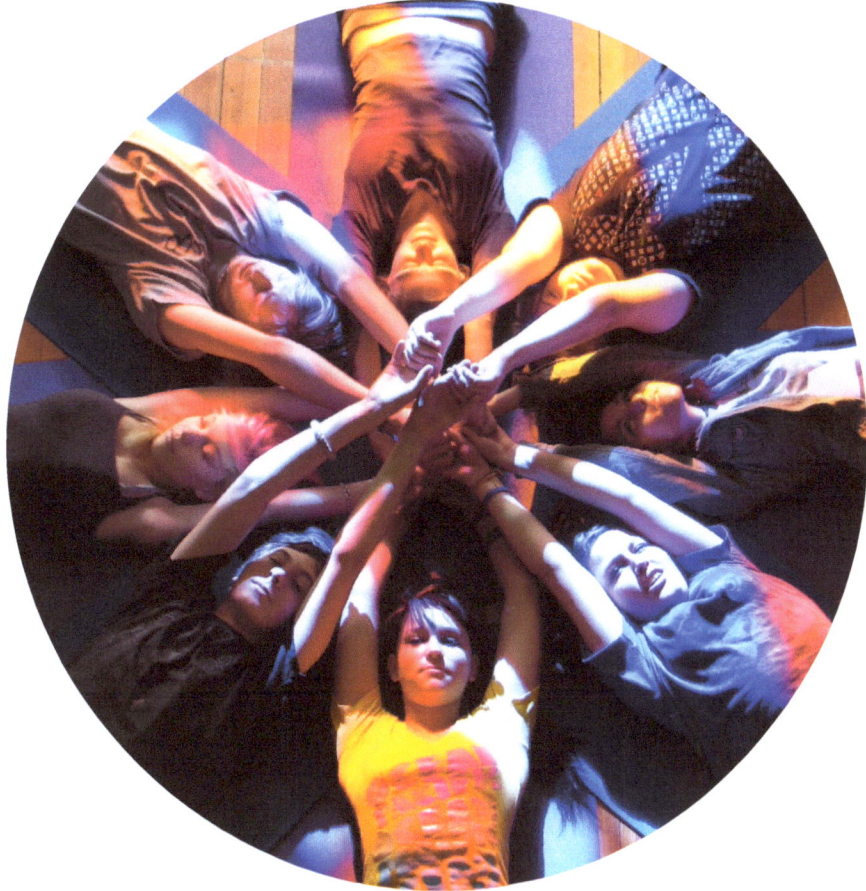

INTRODUCTION

Mandala Yoga is a wonderful way to combine *movement* with *teamwork* and *learning* with *fun*! If you can find space and a group of willing participants, you have all you need. This book provides simple instructions and photographs to serve as a guide so that you are able to visualize each step to create the final pose.

A mandala is a circle, a circumference with a center point, which contains *possibility!* You are invited to explore the idea of a mandala through movement, to become part of an intertwined circle with others, to experience group dynamics and teamwork, and to stretch and strengthen in both body and mind. The mandala poses are fun and accessible for people of all ages. In addition to the multiple health benefits of yoga, there is also a sense of magic that occurs when a group of people work together toward a common goal. You do not need to be super fit or flexible to experience Mandala Yoga. Most of the poses require simple movements, which are supported by proper placement rather than muscles. The book is organized so that the more challenging poses are found toward the end, so you can build in strength, flexibility, and coordination over time. Make a circle and let the fun begin!

WE ARE ALL CONNECTED. WE ARE A MANDALA.

FOUNDATION POSES

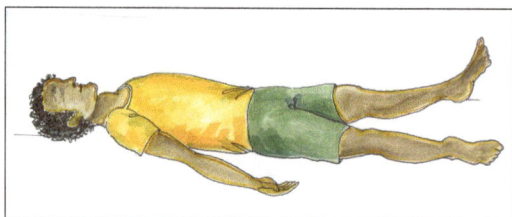

RESTING POSE:

Lie on your back with your palms facing upward and allow the feet to fall comfortably away from each other. Let your body completely relax, from the bottom of your feet to the crown of your head. See if you can feel the very center of the back of your head as it presses into the ground. Beginning at the back of the neck, follow the curves of your spine downward, through the shoulders and middle back, to the tip of the tailbone. Feel that your body is aligned against the support of the floor. Breathe and let your body go limp.

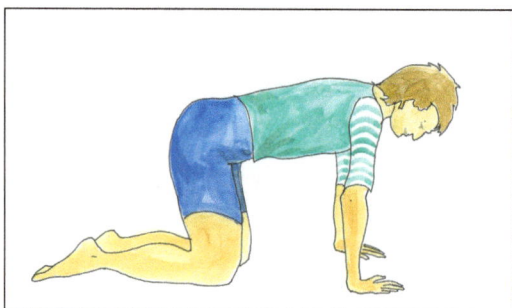

TABLE POSITION:

Any posture that begins on hands and knees begins in Table Position. As with all foundation poses, proper alignment is very important. Begin on hands and knees, with the hands directly beneath the shoulders, your palms flat on the floor, and your fingers open wide. The knees are hip-distance apart and underneath the hips. Lengthen through the spine for a flat back (like a table). Keep the neck aligned with the spine.

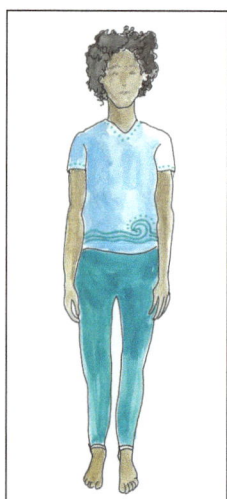

MOUNTAIN POSE:

Stand with your feet hip distance apart and spread your toes out like the roots of a tree. See if you can feel all four corners of your feet as they press into the ground. This is your foundation. Point your tailbone toward the floor, and imagine a string attached from the center of your head to the ceiling. Pull your shoulder blades down the back. Let your arms hang at your sides and draw the shoulders down away from your ears. Feel the weight at your fingertips. Mountain Pose is used to cultivate awareness and stillness. Any pose that begins in standing begins in Mountain Pose in order to center the body and bring the self into alignment, both mentally and physically.

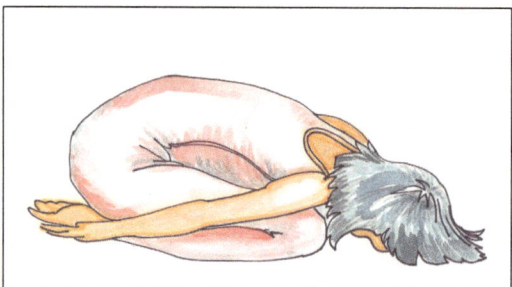

CHILD'S POSE:

From Table Position, move the hips back so that your sitz bones move toward the heels. Fold your upper body down over the knees and rest the forehead on the floor. Let the shoulders round as you take several deep breaths. This pose rejuvenates the whole body as it relaxes your back and stretches the spine.

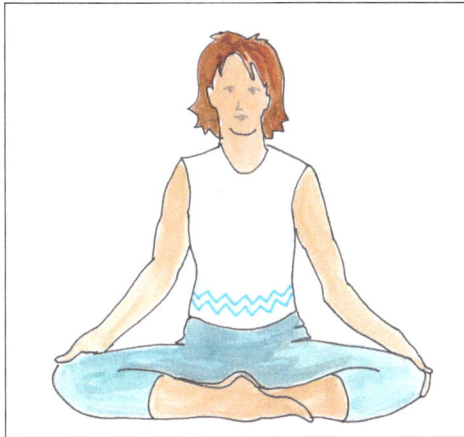

Easy Sit Pose:

Sit with legs crossed in front of you. The sole of the inside foot rests against the inner thigh, while the sole of the outside foot rests against the outside of the shin. Sitting directly on your sitz bones, imagine there is a string attached from the top of your head to the ceiling, suspending the skull and aligning each vertebra. Feel the bones of your spine as they stack up on top of one another, supporting your skull and entire body. The very base of the spine, the tailbone, is pointing downward and anchored into the ground.

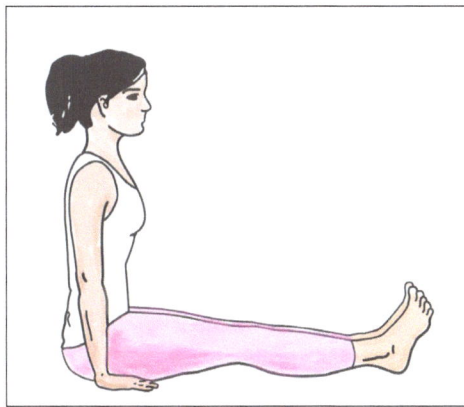

Staff Pose:

Sit on the floor with your legs extended straight in front of you. Align your feet so that they are hip-width apart. Point your toes up toward the sky, and then pull them back toward your nose to activate the muscles in your legs. Roll the thighs inward until the kneecaps face the sky, and place your palms just behind your hips with the fingers pointing towards your feet. Press your palms gently into the ground. Lift into the crown and lengthen through the spine.

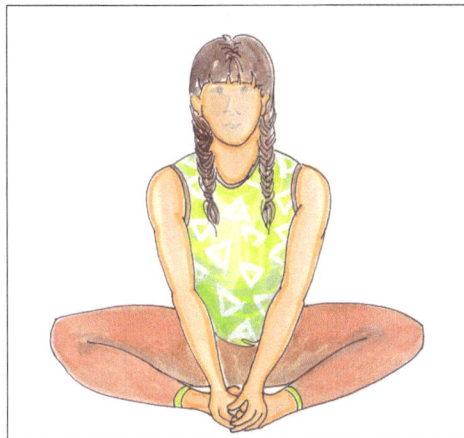

Butterfly Pose:

Sit directly on the sitz bones with the soles of the feet together and the knees open wide. Lift into the crown of the head and drop the shoulders away from the ears. Feel a stretch in your inner thigh muscles.

3

Secondary Poses

Plank Pose:

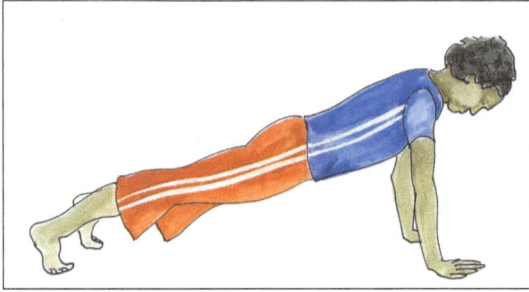

Begin in Table position. Outstretch your right leg behind you, pressing the ball mount of the big toe into the ground. When you feel balanced, repeat the same actions for the left leg and foot. Be sure to raise your hips so that they are not collapsing; as you do so, firm your legs. Relax your shoulders down the back, and lengthen your tailbone towards your feet. Your body makes a diagonal line from head to foot and your arms, chest, core, and leg muscles are strongly engaged.

Downward-facing Dog:

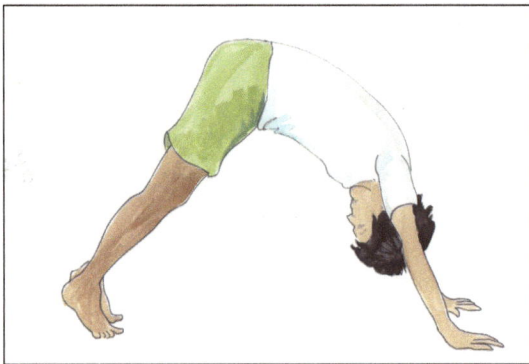

Begin in Table position. As you exhale, lift your knees away from the floor. Keep the knees bent slightly as you lengthen your tailbone away from the back of the pelvis and lift your sitting bones toward the ceiling. As you inhale, push the hamstrings back, roll your thighs inward, and stretch your heels toward the floor. Straighten your knees, but do not lock them. Firm the outer arms and press the pads of your fingers into the floor. See if you can widen your shoulder blades and bring them down the back, toward the tailbone. Keep your head between the upper arms and relax your neck.

Plow Pose:

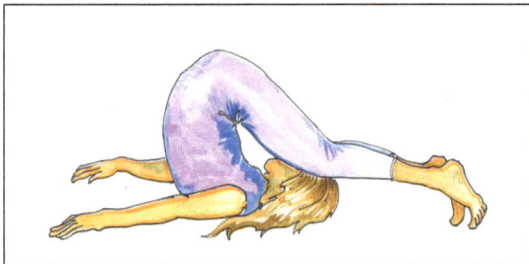

Begin in Resting Pose. Bend your knees, bringing your feet to the floor with the heels close to your hips. On an exhalation, press your arms into the ground as you push your feet away from the ground and bring your thighs to the top of your chest. As you inhale, continue to lift your legs by curling your back torso and pelvis away from the ground as your knees move toward your face. Bring your palms to your lower back, or extend your arms against the ground. As you exhale, slowly extend first one leg and then the other out straight, with your toes on the ground if possible.(Your legs are now behind your head.) Take care not to turn your head from side to side here. Remove your hands from your back and stretch your arms out straight, bringing your palms flat to the floor. Clasp your hands together as your raise your hips, push into the toes, and pull the shoulder blades away from the back.

** TO EXIT THE POSE: Carefully lift one leg at a time until both legs are straight in the air. Slowly drop the tailbone back to the ground and bend your knees so that they rest on your chest. Take some deep breaths here. Lower your feet to the ground, keeping your knees bent, and allow your spine to rest here for a few moments.

MANDALA YOGA POSES

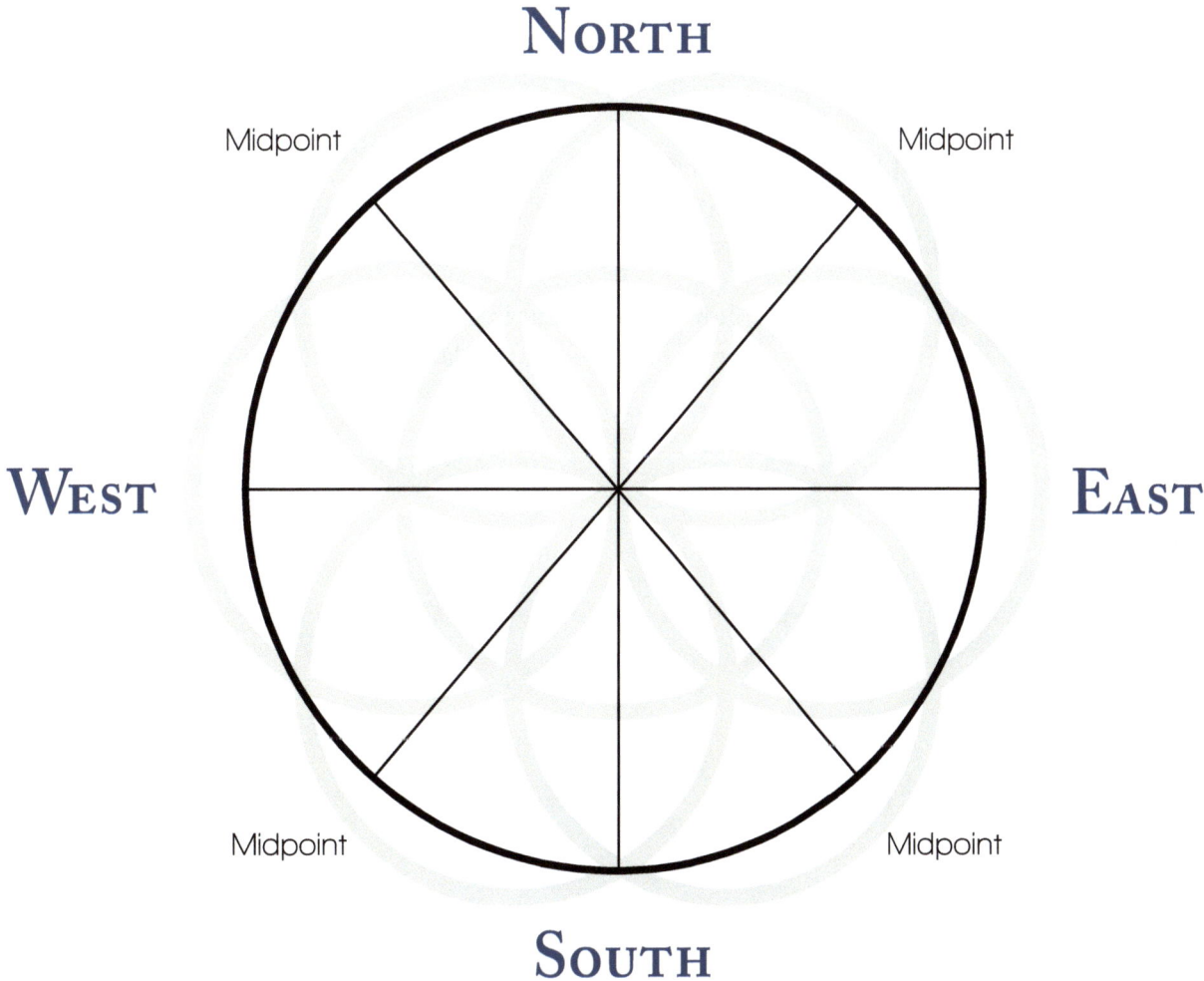

NORTH

Midpoint   Midpoint

WEST   **EAST**

Midpoint   Midpoint

SOUTH

THE FOUR DIRECTIONS

This pose requires eight people divided into two teams of four.

MOVEMENT INSTRUCTIONS:

~ Team 1: Participants are arranged in a seated position, facing North/South and East/West. Spines are lifted with the legs straight toward the center of the circle in Staff Pose. Hands rest, palms down, on the knees.

~ Team 2: Participants sit in between the four directions (the midpoints) and lie down on their backs with arms extended up by the ears, creating one long line with the body.

> ** All eight practitioners should align their feet toward the center to form an inner circle.*

~ As Team 1 slowly lifts their arms, they roll down each vertebra until they are lying flat on their backs. Simultaneously, participants in Team 2 engage their abdominal muscles and slowly roll up their spines until they are in a seated Staff Pose.

* Both teams should coordinate the movement so that it happens simultaneously. The synchronization of the movement is challenging and places a strong emphasis on teamwork.

> ** Repeat several times to practice attaining a perfect synchronized movement.*

> ** For a greater meditative effect, each practitioner can attune the breath with the movement: Inhale-up, Exhale-down.*

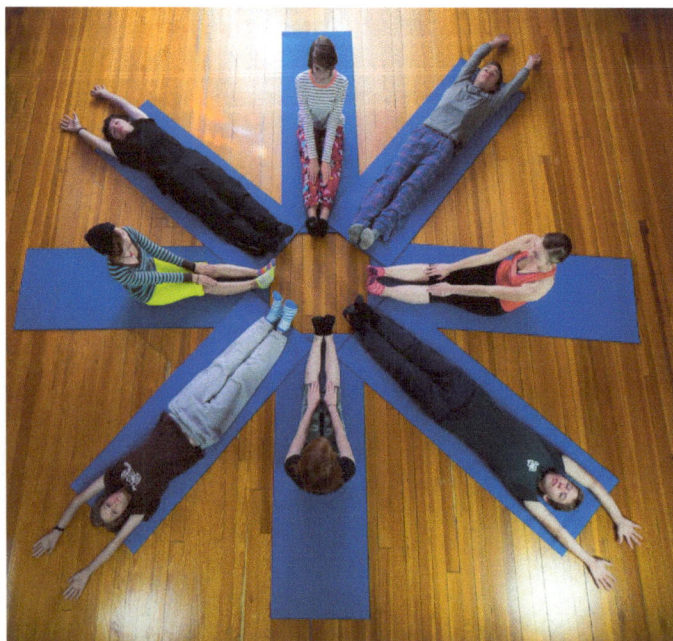

KING'S CROWN

This pose requires eight people divided into two teams of four.

MOVEMENT INSTRUCTIONS:

~ Eight practitioners (Teams 1 and 2) form a circle and sit in Staff Pose, each person facing the center with the feet nearly touching.

~ Team 1 consists of those practitioners who are facing the four directions. Practitioners roll down their spines to recline in resting pose. Now draw the knees up and the feet off the floor. Connect the feet around the four directions.

~ Team 2 (the midpoints) lie down with their knees bent and feet flat on the floor.

~ Team 2 brings the feet up off the floor to connect above Team 1. Now Team 2 can straighten the legs to form a circle of "V"s.

> ** The lifted legs should feel supported by the weight of your neighbors' legs leaning into yours.*

~ All practitioners open their arms wide and connect arms at the elbows with their neighbors to complete the outside circle.

~ Switch teams and perform the actions of the pose again.

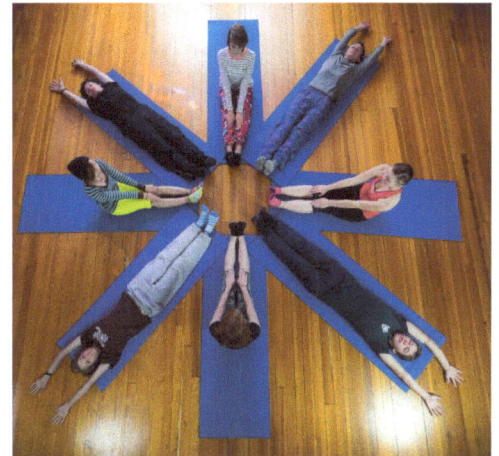

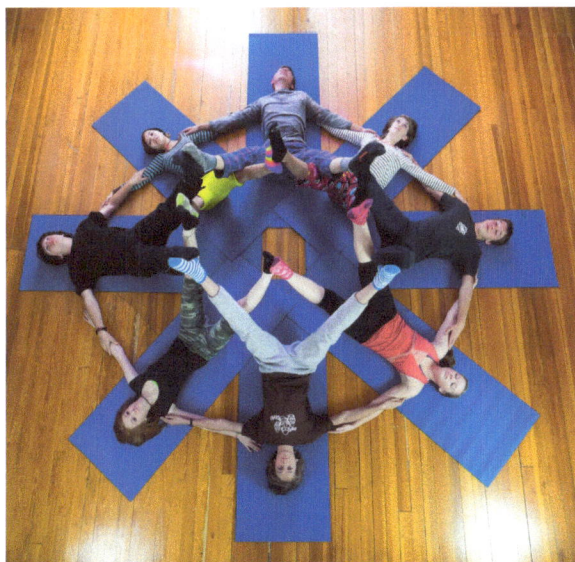

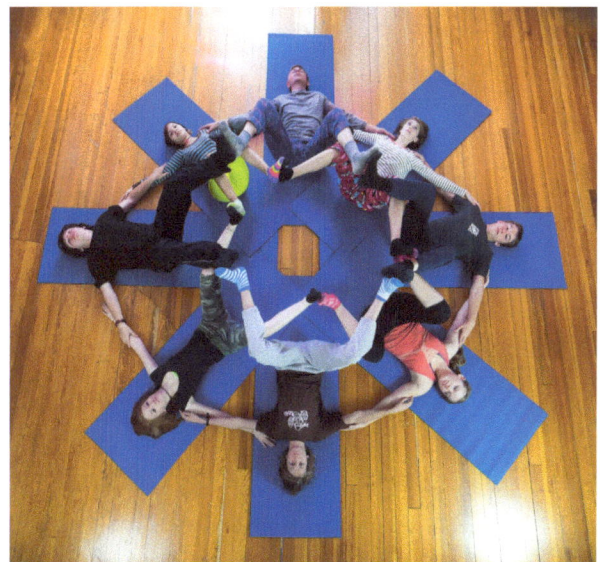

OCTOPUS

This pose is best suited for eight people but can be done with any even number of people, up to ten.

MOVEMENT INSTRUCTIONS:

~ Participants lie down in resting pose with the heads toward the center of the circle.

~ Participants reach their arms backward and over their heads, then connect hands with the person directly opposite in the circle.

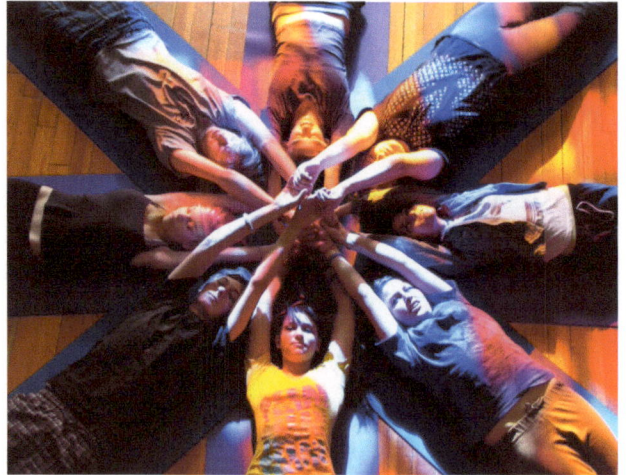

~ Utilizing the connection at the hands for stability, each practitioner lifts both legs straight up toward the sky. Be sure to keep the pelvis anchored to the ground.

* This action requires a good amount of core strength.

* Movements should be synchronized with the other practitioners.

* Coordinate your breath so that you exhale as you lift the legs. Remember that proper breathing helps to increase your strength.

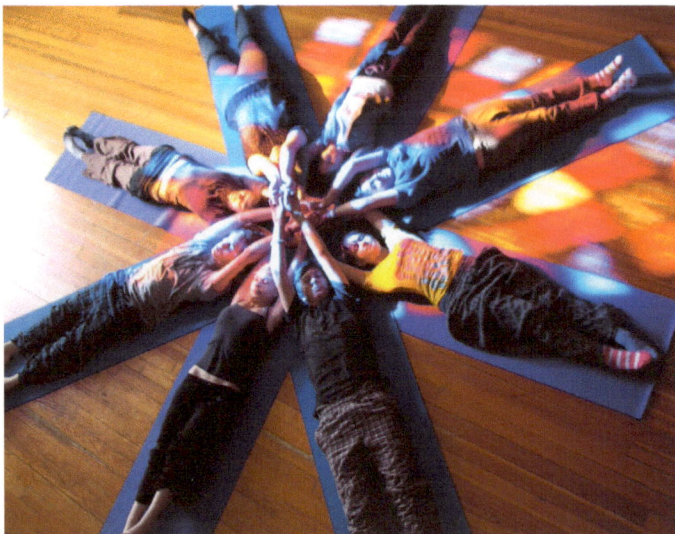

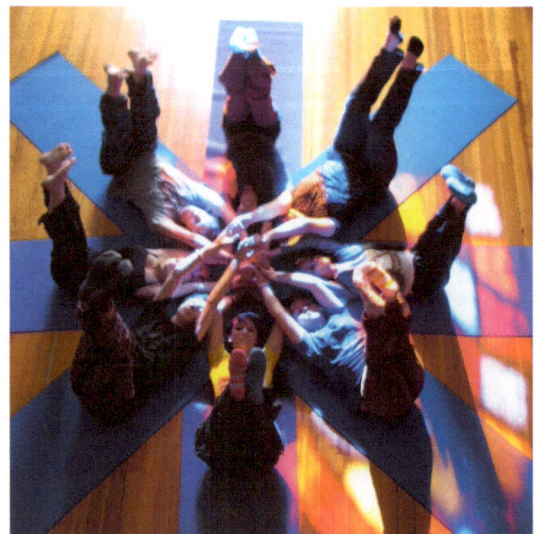

BICYCLE WHEEL

This pose is best suited for eight people but can be done with any even number of people, up to ten.

MOVEMENT INSTRUCTIONS:

~ From the starting position of Octopus, each practitioner simultaneously lifts the left leg, allowing the right leg to rest straight out on the floor.

~ Slowly lower the lifted left leg down, across the midline of the body and over the right hip.

> ** This is a good twist for the torso. Take several deep breaths, which will help to massage the internal organs.*

~ Lift the left leg back up to center and repeat the movement with the right leg crossing over to the left side of the body.

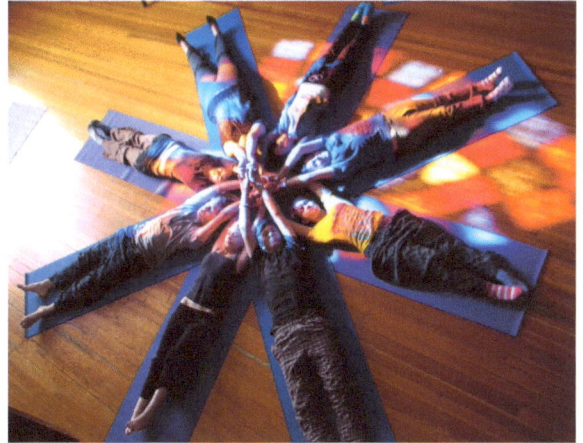

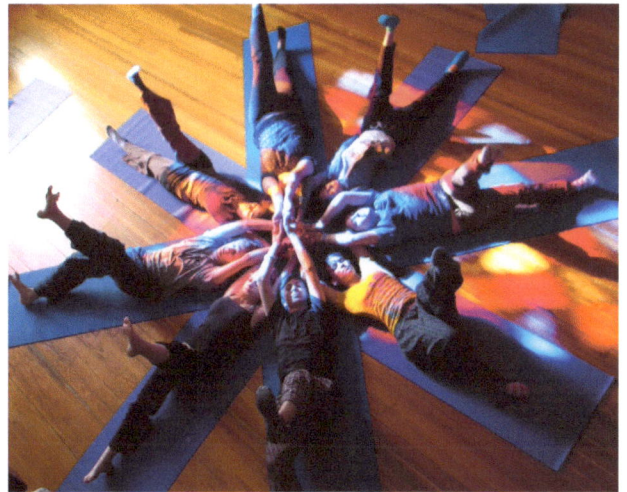

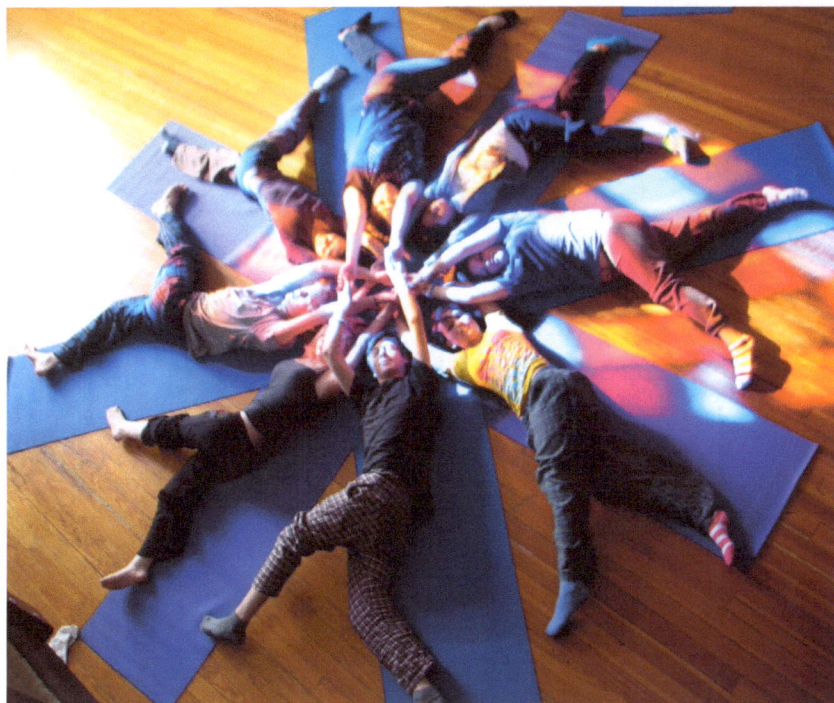

SIMPLE FLOWER

This pose requires eight people divided into two teams of four.

MOVEMENT INSTRUCTIONS:

~ Begin this pose with eight practitioners lying on their backs, alternating head and feet toward the center of the circle.

~ Each practitioner brings their arms out at a 45 degree angle.

~ The people lying in the four directions (Team 1) rest their hands face down in the open palms of their Team 2 partner.

~ Practitioners touch their thumbs together lightly with their neighbors' thumbs.

* The arms, once connected, create the petals of a simple flower.

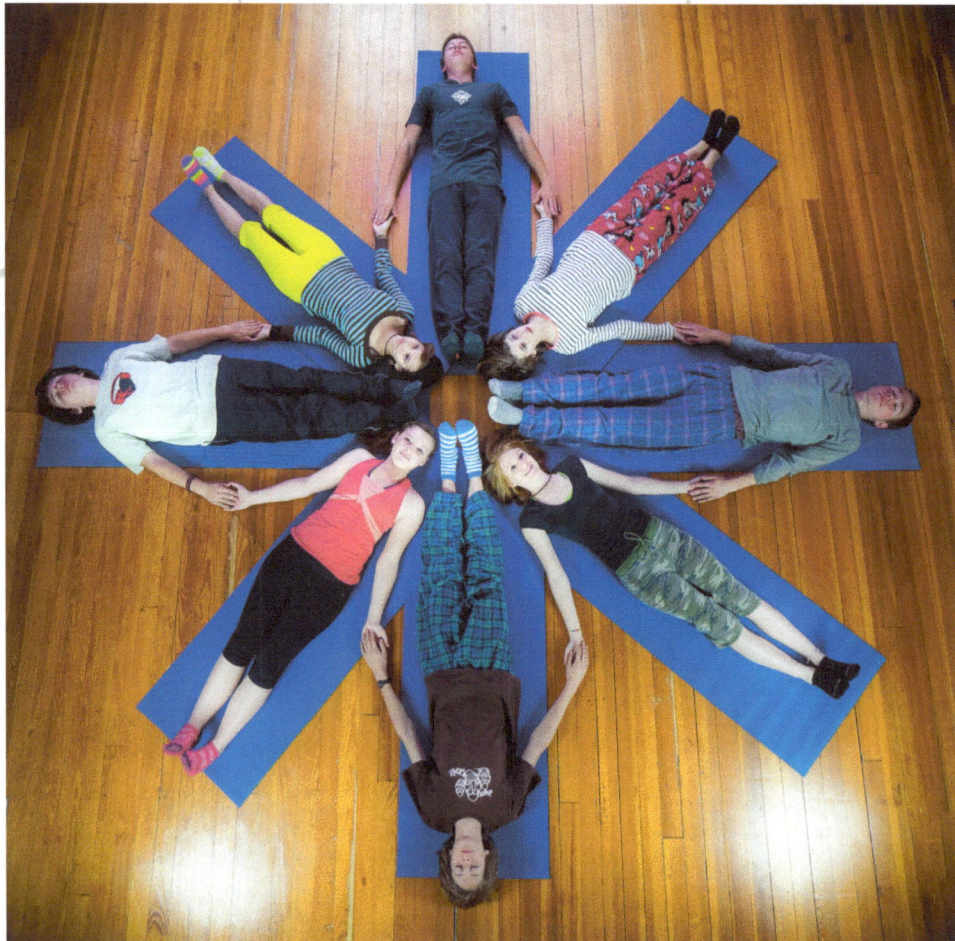

QUEEN'S CROWN

This design requires eight people but can be done with 10 people. This makes the leg span a shorter distance.

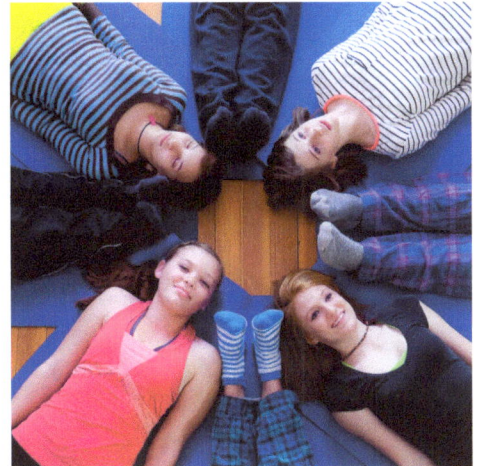

MOVEMENT INSTRUCTIONS:

* When planning this mandala, see that those with more flexibility have their feet pointing out. Participants with feet pointing out in the circle will have a wider span to open their legs.

~ Start in Simple Flower with eight people lying in a circle, alternating head and feet toward the center.

~ Each participant raises their arms up straight, toward the sky, with hands open.

* The hands will receive the partners' ankles on the next move.

~ Participants raise their legs (one leg at a time is easier for beginners) and place their ankles in the open hands of their neighbors.

* Once all legs are up, this pose should be completely supported and easy to hold. Make sure the arms are outstretched and straight to support the weight of the legs.

* If you would like to turn this pose into a strengthening pose, use the muscle energy of the arms to lift and lower the legs, like a bench press.

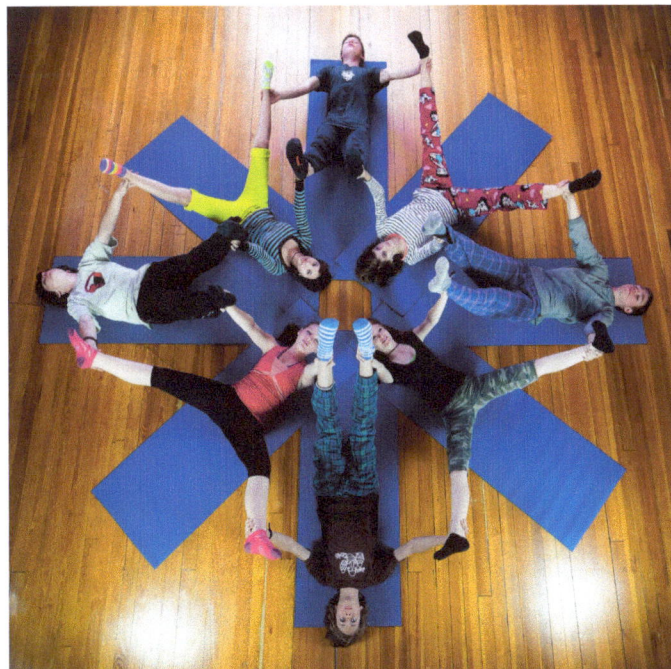

VENUS FLY TRAP

This pose can be accomplished with a minimum of four people.

MOVEMENT INSTRUCTIONS:

~ Four participants sit facing each other toward the center of the circle.

~ All four participants bend their knees and place the soles of their feet on the floor.

~ North/South participants bring the balls of their feet together. These two participants lie down on their backs, push into their partner's feet and, with knees bent at a right angle, bring the feet up off the floor.

~ The other two participants (East/West) repeat the same actions of the North/South participants.

> ** One pair of feet is nestled between the other pair of feet.*

~ All four people now clasp hands or arms to connect the circle.

~ Each participant now straightens his/her legs. Keep contact with your partner's feet by imagining yours are stuck to theirs with glue.

~ In the final step of this pose, all four participants simultaneously open the legs wide and then close them.

> ** Repeat the last action several times to ensure smooth movement.*

> ** This pose strengthens the abdominal muscles and provides a nice stretch for the inner thigh muscles.*

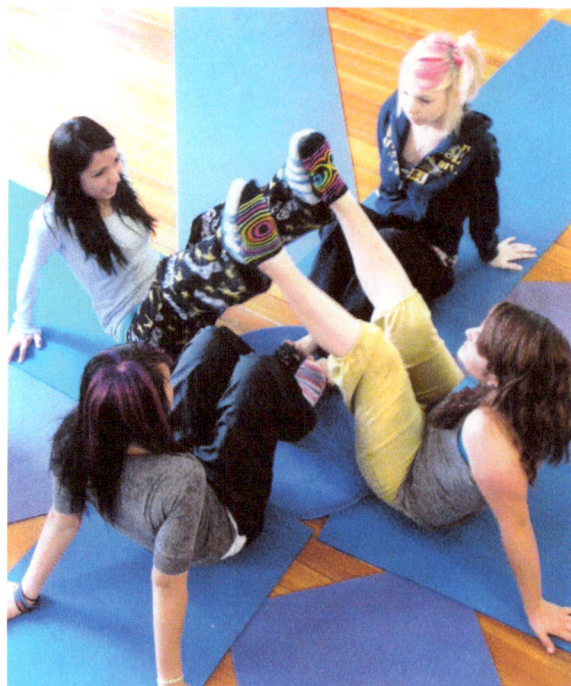

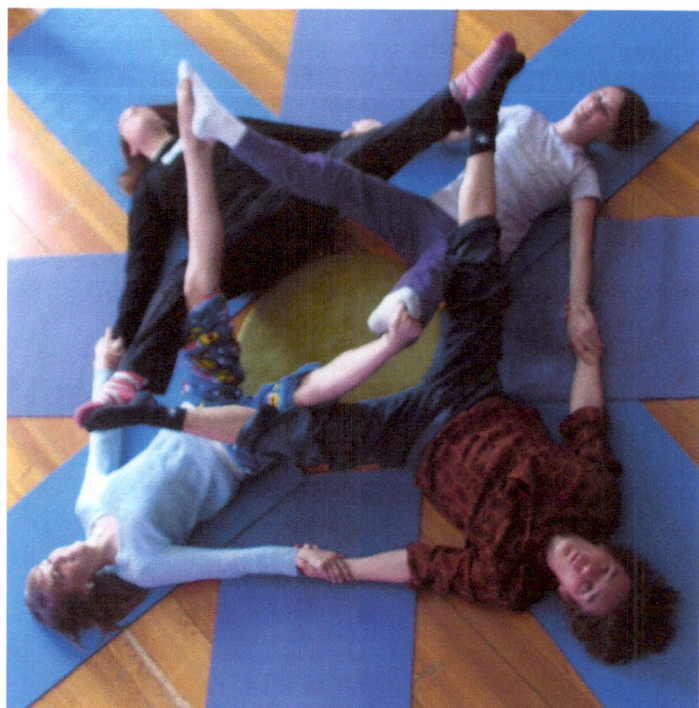

12

CREAM PUFF

This design requires four people, but can be done with more people.

MOVEMENT INSTRUCTIONS:

~ Begin with all practitioners lying on their backs in the four directions with their heads toward the center.

~ Everyone should have their legs bent, feet flat, with arms by their sides on the floor.

~ Bring the knees in toward your chest and straighten your legs toward the ceiling.

~ Now lower the legs toward the center one person at a time. Use the arms to push into the floor for more stability.

~ Each participants feet should stack over the next, creating a deep stretch for the one that is on the bottom of the stack.

> ** Take turns being the one on the bottom of the stack.*
>
> ** Placement of the heads is important: when everyone rolls back into Plow Pose, the legs are outstretched and the soles of the feet meet in the middle.*
>
> ** Be sure not to move the neck from side to side in this pose.*
>
> ** If adjustments need to be made, take the time to make them before beginning again.*

~Finally, everyone connects arms around the circle.

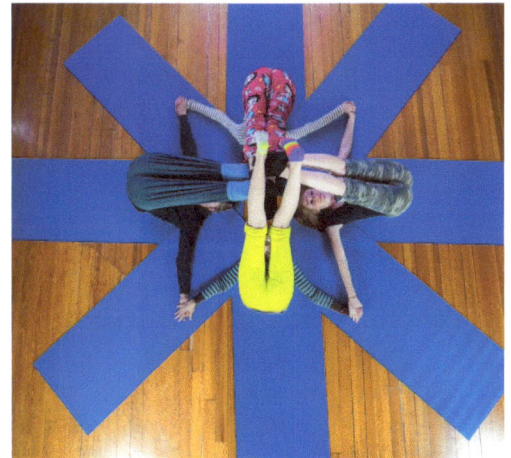

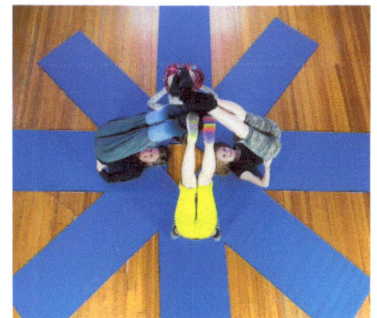

VARIATION

Use your hands placed on the lower back to hold yourself up and lift up onto the shoulders. Keep the legs straight, and toes meet in the middle.

VARIATION

From Plow pose, bend the knees and draw them together toward the center of the body, while bringing the feet out, in the direction of your neighbors. Touch feet.

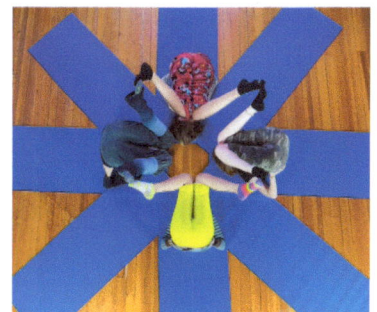

SEA STAR

This design requires eight people, but can be done with more.

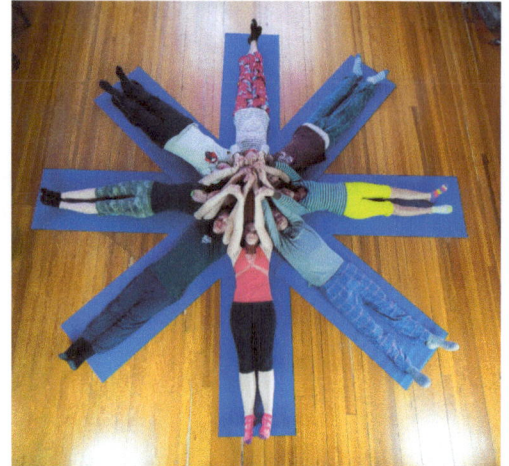

MOVEMENT INSTRUCTIONS:

~ All participants begin by lying on their backs with their heads toward the center of the circle. The legs are outstretched and the feet are relaxed.

~ Every other person, Team 1 (four directions) raises his/her arms toward the sky and joins hands with the alternating neighbors.

~ The other participants, Team 2 (midpoints) whose arms are down, connect their hands with their alternating neighbors.

~ Team 1 bring the raised arms down to rest on the lower set of adjoined arms.

   * Arms should be relaxed with the connected hands resting on the belly. Notice the beautiful flower that is formed with the arms.

~ As you slowly inhale, all practitioners straighten their interconnected arms.

~ Exhale Lift both sets of arms.

~ As participants raise both sets of arms up to the sky, all hands meet in the center.

~ Inhale in the center

~ Exhale and lower the arms.

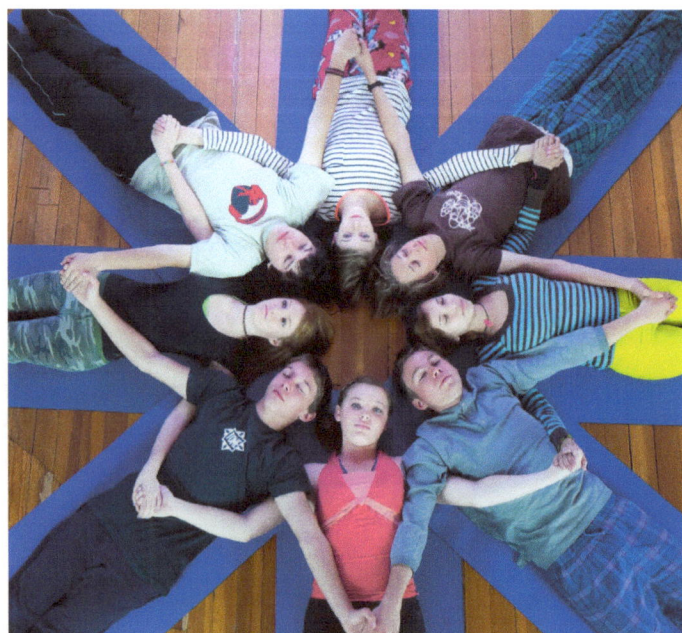

Sea Star Continued

~ Inhale, using the abdominal muscles to raise both legs and feet to the sky.

~ Exhale, lowering the legs to the ground.

> *You can bend the legs as you lift, if necessary. Eventually, your abdominal muscles will be strong enough to lift the legs straight to the sky.*
>
> *Coordinating the movement to move the arms and legs simultaneously is fun.*

~ End the pose by bringing the legs toward the floor into Butterfly Pose (soles of the feet together with knees open as wide as possible).

~Relax and feel the breath of everyone in the circle.

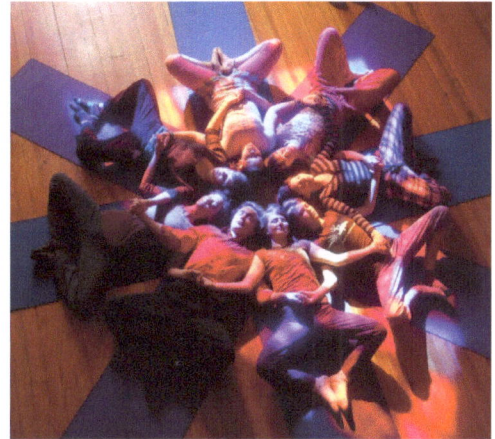

Variation

Legs connect, the same way the arms did. One team at a time, lift the legs and connect feet in the air.

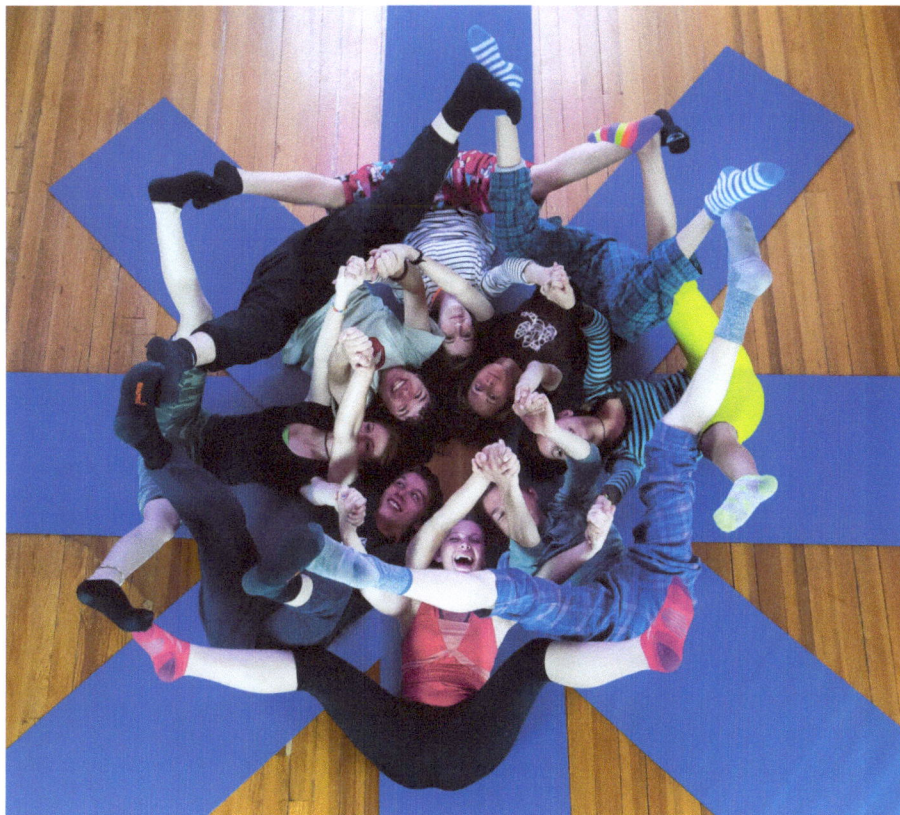

Folding Flower

This design requires six or eight people but can be done with any even number of people.

Movement Instructions:

~ As practitioners stand in Mountain Pose in a circle, each person places a hand on the lower back of both neighbors.

~ In unison, everyone hinges forward from the waist. Come to a right angle with the spine straight and elongated.

~ Keep the eyes on the floor and the neck aligned with the extended spine.

~ Hold for several breaths.

~ Simultaneously, everybody folds forward toward the floor, releasing the neck and head completely.

~ Bend and straighten the knees. Play with synchronizing this movement and coordinating the breath with the motion of the body.

~ As a team, bend the knees and roll up the spine slowly to the initial standing position.

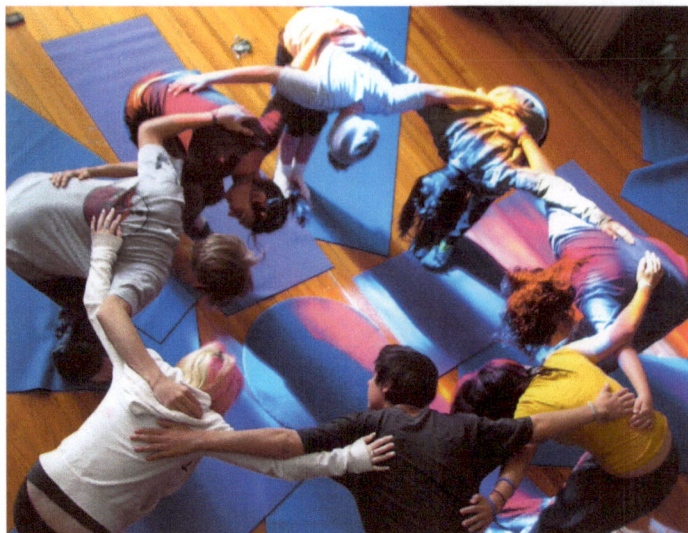

Variation I

Fold the torso in the opposite other direction, arching the back and clasping the hands to support the opening of the chest toward the sky. This variation takes teamwork, balance, and trust. It is more challenging and therefore, takes time to achieve.

Variation II

Another way to begin this variation is for alternating persons to arch back while those in between stand straight and serve as support.

* This is an excercise in trust!

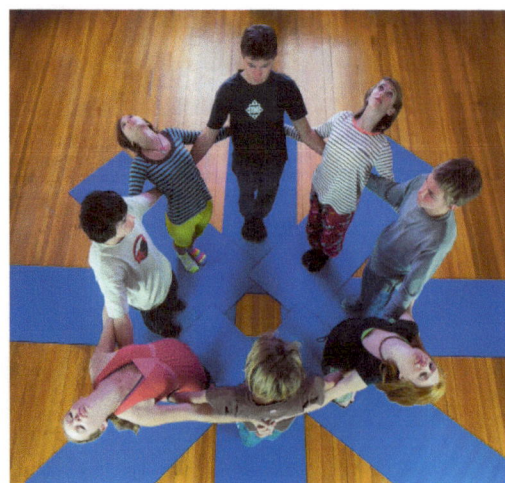

EXPLODING STAR

This design requires five people, but can be done with more people.

MOVEMENT INSTRUCTIONS:

~ All five practitioners begin standing and facing the center of the circle.

~ Bring the arms straight forward, shoulder-height, and rotate the arms so that the palms face out.

~ Each person's hands will be palm-to-palm with the people on either side of them.

~ Keeping the arms straight out in front of the body, bring the arms up and around slowly until the arms are in a T-shaped position. This movement rotates the arms in the sockets. As you open your arms, take a step back.

~ Make sure the thumbs point up to the sky and the finger tips point out.

~ With the arms in a T-position, take one step inward to create the star. As you push into your neighbors' palms gently, you will feel a stretch in the pectoral muscles in the chest.

* Keep a strong connection between the palms of the hands throughout the movement.

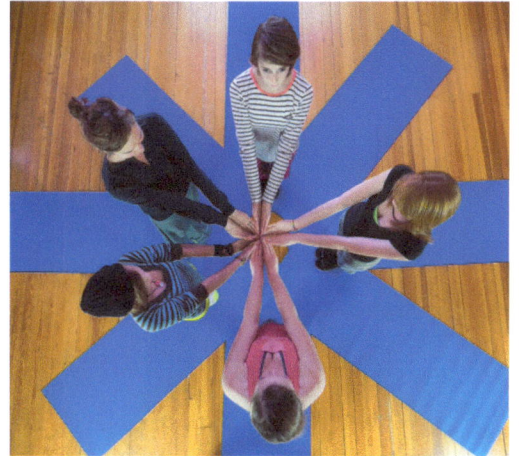

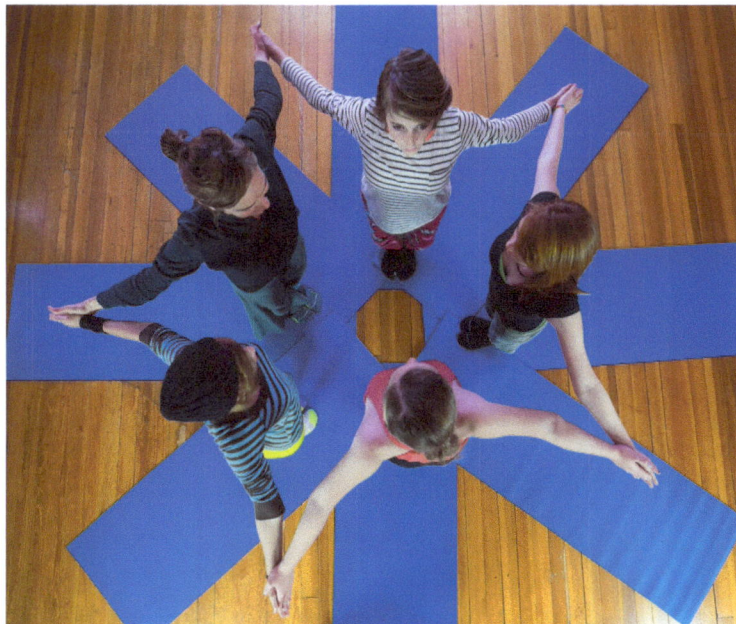

GEOMETRIC ARM WAVE

This design requires six people divided into two teams of three. This pose can be done with more people.

MOVEMENT INSTRUCTIONS:

~ Begin by standing in a circle. Visually divide into two teams (one even team, one odd team). The "even" team clasps hands with each other, arms in the air. The "odd" team then clasps hands with each other, arms down low. Bring both sets of clasped hands down inside the circle. This will create two separate circles of hands: an upper circle and a lower circle.

~ The members of both circles keep arms clasped and bring the arms forward, up and over head and all the way around to the back.

> ** The connected arms revolve from the front, over the head, and behind the back.*

~ In unison, lean back, keeping the body extended at a diagonal line, and find balance. Everyone should be supporting everyone else.

> ** Complete the actions of this pose several times to create fluid movements.*

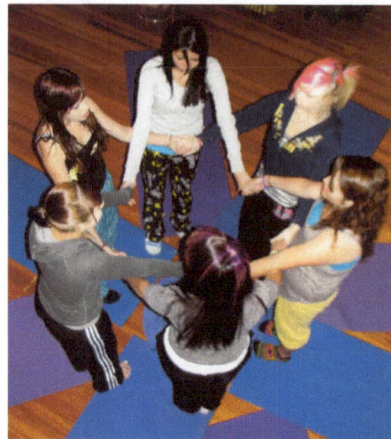

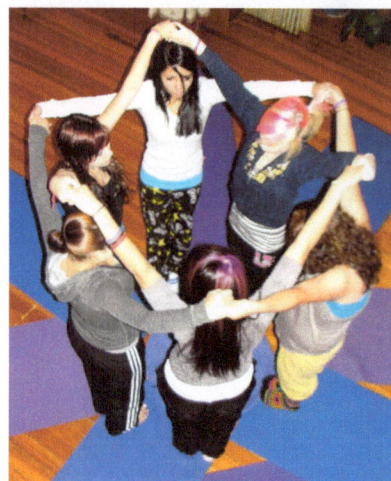

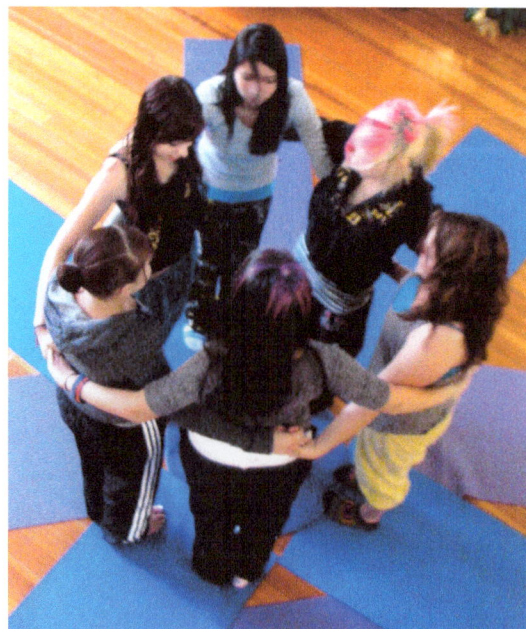

VARIATION

Every other person leans back, arching the spine, into a supported back bend.

Celtic Triangle

This pose requires three people.

Movement instructions:

~ Participants stand facing each other.

~ Hold each other's arms just above the elbows to establish balance and connection.

> *This is the first of two triangles in this pose.*

~ One participant begins the second triangle by bending his/her left leg and bringing the left foot on to their own right thigh. This creates a landing on which the second person's foot will rest.

~ The second participant brings his/her left leg up straight and rests the foot on the top of the first person's right thigh.

~ The third participant brings his/her left leg up straight and rests the foot on the second person's right thigh.

~ Finally, the first person unbends his/her "landing" leg, straightens it, and rests it on the third person's thigh. All three people are now standing balanced on the right leg.

> *The legs create the second triangle in this pose.*
>
> *This pose requires flexible hamstrings!*
>
> *This pose may feel unbalanced at first, but once all steps are completed, it should feel very balanced.*
>
> *When finished, always remember to do the pose standing on the opposite leg as a way to balance the body.*

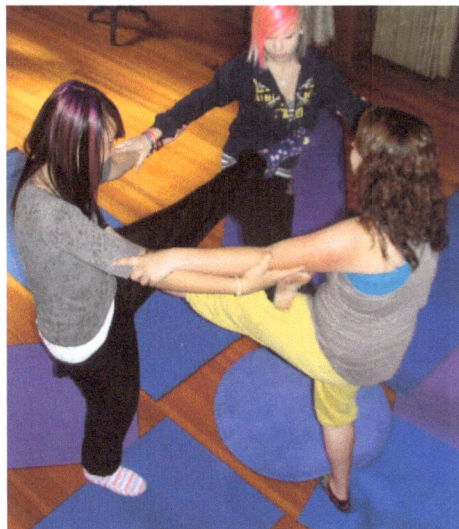

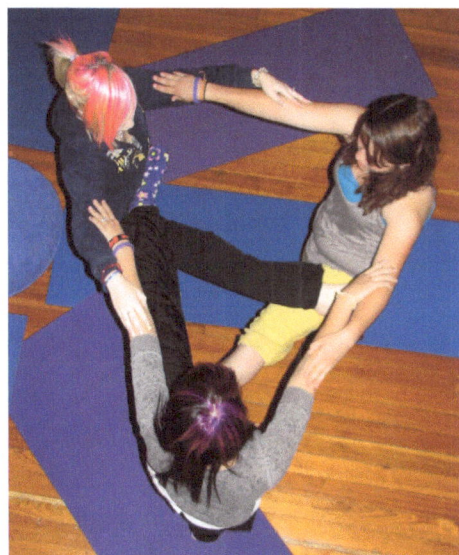

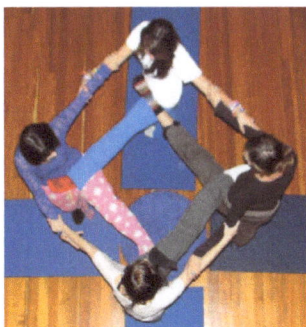

Celtic Square

This actions of this pose are the same as the Celtic Triangle. The difference is that this pose, done with four people, creates a square.

Downward-Facing Dog
Upward-Facing Dog Flow

This flow can be done with any even number of people.

Movement Instructions:

~ Begin so that all participants are in Table Position, alternating with every other person facing outwards.

*The four directions face in and the midpoints face out.

~ From Table Position, move into Plank Pose: lengthen the legs fully and push into the toes, bringing the knees off the ground. Participants are balanced on the hands and balls of the feet with their spines extended straight.

~ From Plank Pose, every other person lifts the pelvis up and points the tailbone toward the ceiling into Downward-facing Dog Pose.

~ Simultaneously, the alternate practitioners drop the pelvis down, coming into upward-facing Dog.

~ On the count of three, everyone slowly moves into the opposite pose.

* You may want to count as the transition takes place (one group lifting the pelvis while the other group drops the pelvis) so that the movements are coordinated.

* It may take some practice to achieve group coordination. You can also work with coordinating the breath: inhale into Upward-facing Dog and exhale into Downward-facing Dog.

* Once you achieve the pose fully, you can play with variations by adding more poses to the flow.

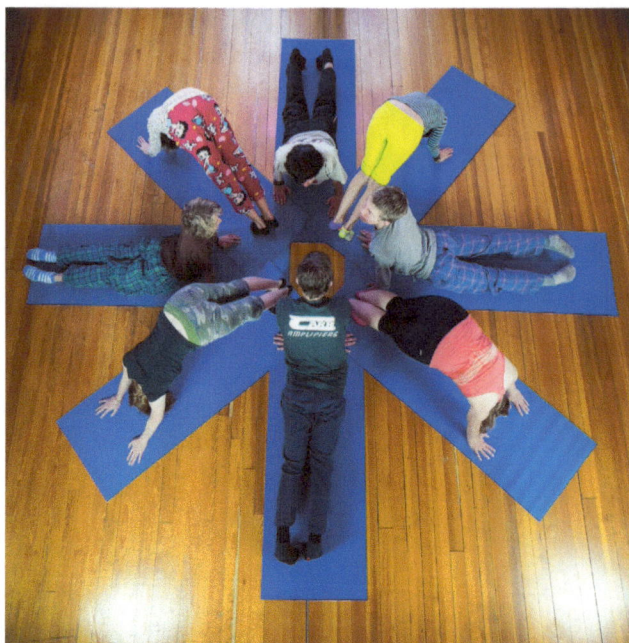

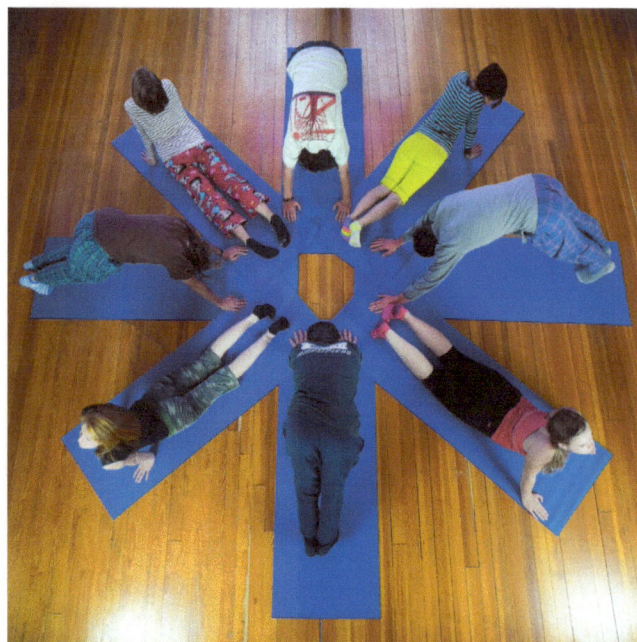

Variation on Downward-Facing Dog
Upward-Facing Dog Flow

This flow can be done with any even number of people.

Movement Instructions:

Add in warrior pose,

~ All participants meet in Plank pose and then draw the left foot forward in between the hands (lunge).

~From the lunge, push into the foot and rise up into the warrior pose. Connect every other hand throughout the circle (hands will be connected behind each other's back).

~ Now straighten the front leg and lean forward with a flat back.

*Use each other for balance!

*This is a strong hamstring stretch.

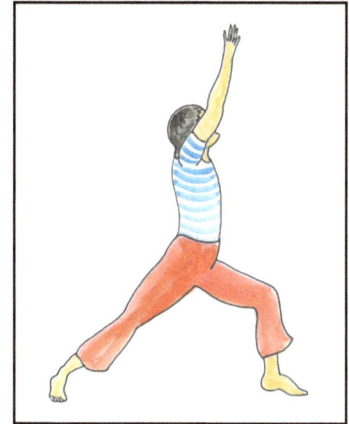

Warrior Pose

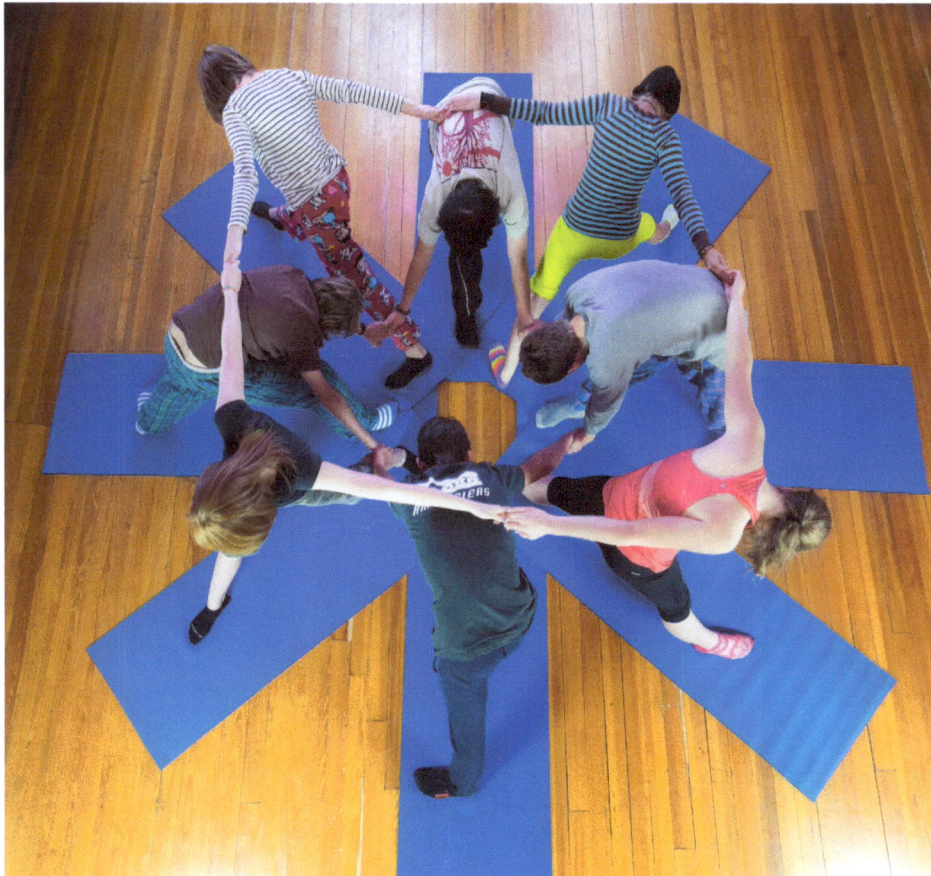

UMBRELLA

This design can be done with anywhere from three to eight people.

MOVEMENT INSTRUCTIONS:

~ Begin in Table Position with heads facing toward the center of the circle.

~ Each person straightens their right leg out behind them, placing the toes and the ball of the foot on the ground for stability.

~ Swivel the left leg like a kick stand, so that the shin is perpendicular to the right leg, and place the shin and ball of the foot on the ground to create a solid foundation. (This action will turn your pelvis and foot toward the right slightly.)

~ Swing the right arm up and over your head toward the center of the circle. Your arm should end up alongside your right ear with the palm facing toward the ground.

> ** The left arm and leg support you as your body, in one line from the right finger to the right toes, creates a long side body stretch.*

~ The hands in the center of the circle pile on top of one another to create a center connection.

~ Or create a thumb ring!

~ As a group, bring the body back to Table Position slowly and repeat on the other side.

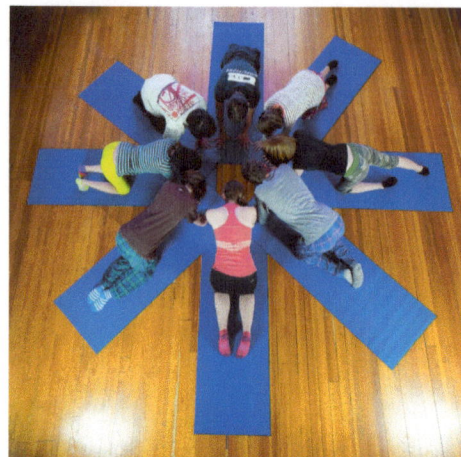

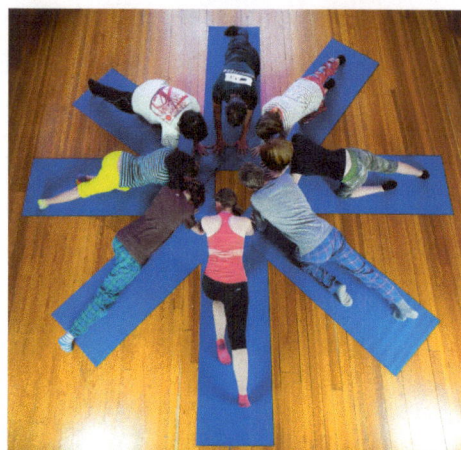

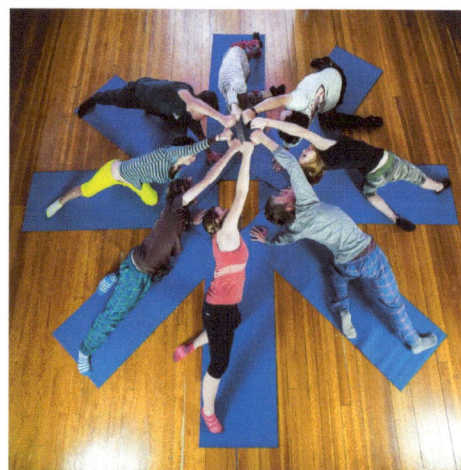

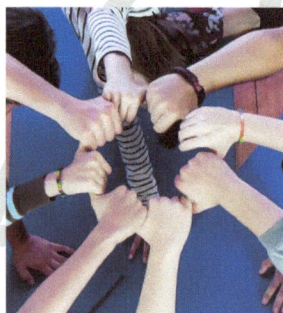

VARIATION

For a more challenging pose, straighten the left leg with the right leg so that the "kick stand" no longer supports the body. Now lift the hips high, using the balancing arm as the only support to the body.

Balancing Cat Flower

This pose works well with eight people, but can be done with fewer; even or odd does not matter.

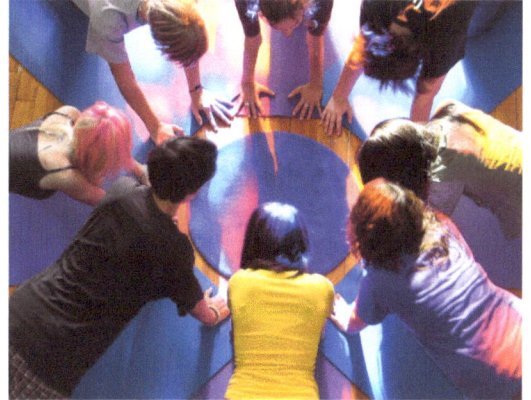

Movement Instructions:

~ Begin with participants on their hands and knees in Table Position, heads facing the center of the circle.

> ** Tables have flat backs, with arms and knees parallel to each other and palms placed firmly on the ground.*

~ Lift the right arm and reach it straight forward, extending completely through the entire right side of the body. Feel how that changes the weight distribution throughout the body. After a stretch, return the arm to the original position.

~ Lift the left leg and extend it out behind you, toes pointed toward the ground. Feel the length of the leg all the way through the left side body. Also, take note of the changes in weight distribution throughout the body. Return the leg to its original position.

~ Now, these two movements are combined: lift the right arm and the left leg simultaneously. Feel the body balance and keep the back flat. Pull the navel back toward the spine to create core strength and integrity in the pose.

~ Come back to Table Position and repeat the previous actions with the opposite arm and leg.

> ** To help maintain balance, use the tip of your extended index finger as a focal point.*

> ** Option: create a Thumb Ring (Page 41) in the center.*

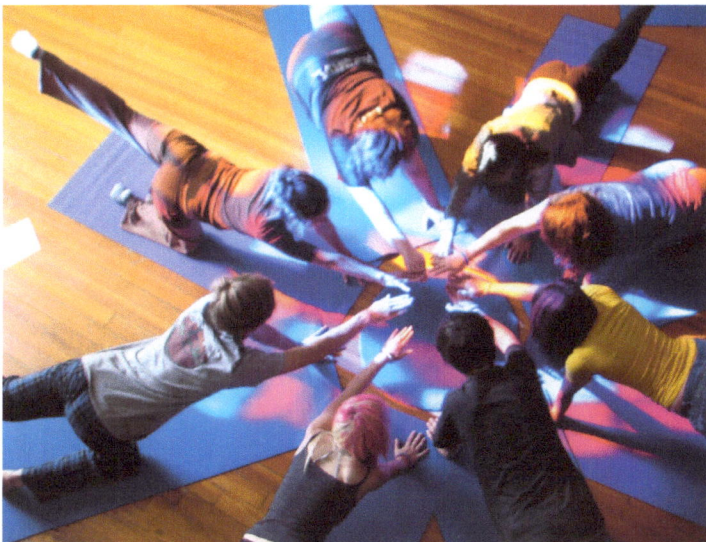

Variation

Place the extended right arm on the left corner of your mat. Next, bring the extended left leg across the mat to the right corner. Place the ball of the foot down. Feel the stretch in the thoracic and lumbar vertebrae of the spine in this variation.

TIGER LILY
VARIATION OF THE BALANCING CAT
FLOWER

This pose works well with eight people, but can be done with six.

MOVEMENT INSTRUCTIONS:

~ Participants are on their hands and knees in Table Position, heads facing the center of the circle.

* Similar to the original pose, except this variation requires every other person begins with opposite arm/leg extended.

* Notice that when you reach across the mat, your hands and legs come together with your neighbors' hands and legs. Accentuate this action to create the effect of a flower petal.

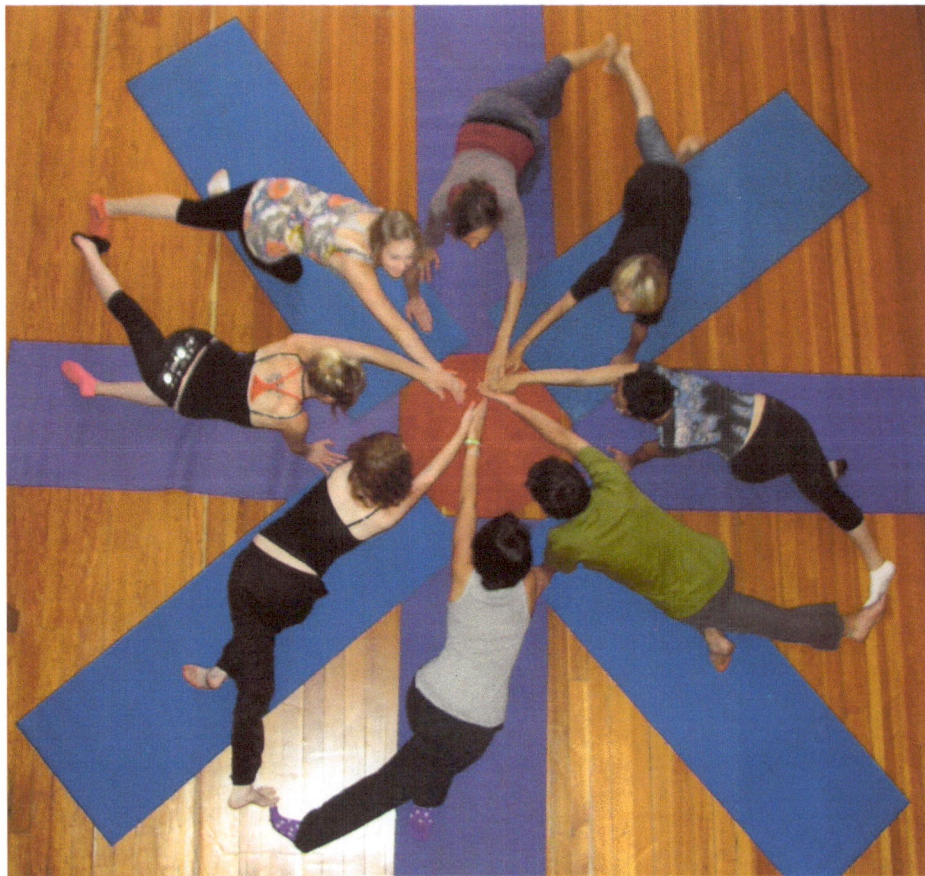

TWISTED VINE

This design requires eight or more people.

MOVEMENT INSTRUCTIONS:

~ Begin with practitioners in Table Position with their heads close together toward the center of the circle.

> ** The positioning in this pose is important. It may take several adjustments to get it right.*

~ From Table Position, bring the left hand through and under the right arm and lay your head on the floor so that it rests on your left ear. Your left arm should rest comfortably on the ground .

~ Breathe and be still here for a moment as you feel the twist and gentle inversion offered by this pose ("Thread the Needle" Pose).

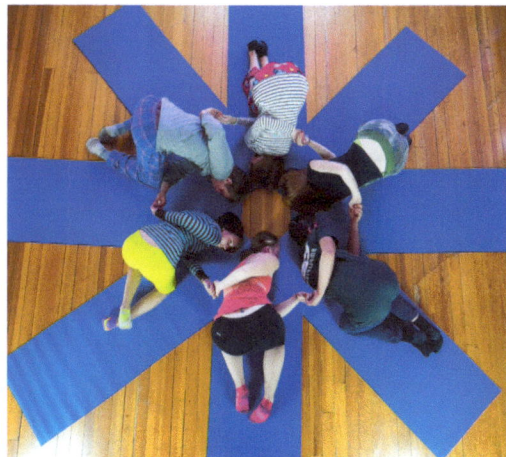

~ Each practitioner raises the right arm toward the sky. Then, bend the right arm at the elbow and bring it down to rest on your lower back.

~ Next, all practioners bend the left arm up to meet the hand of the person in front of you.

~ Take several deep breaths here before unwinding the pose, resting in Table Position for a moment, and repeating the actions of the pose again on the other side of the body. Balancing both sides is important.

THREAD THE NEEDLE POSE

> ** **PROPER POSITIONING IS CRUCIAL!** If the positions are misaligned, you will not be able to clasp hands or you will feel discomfort.*
>
> ** When the position is correct, each practitioner should be able to clasp hands with his/her neighbor in the circle, creating the Twisted Vine and slightly deepening the twist in the torso.*
>
> ** Remember: if at first you don't succeed, try again. That's the fun of it!*
>
> ** Also remember: if your body doesn't feel right, it isn't right. Adjust accordingly. The goal is to stretch and be creative, not to make a design at the expense of your body's comfort.*
>
> ** The most important thing is for the pose to maintain integrity, and once achieved, be sustainable.*

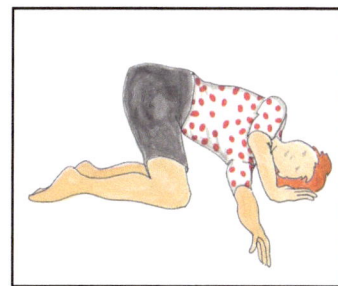

FALLING STAR

This design requires five people, but can be done with any number.

MOVEMENT INSTRUCTIONS:

~ From a seated position with all participants in a circle, turn to face to the right side so that all five participants are now facing the same direction.

~ All five people lie down on their right side.

~ Each person bends their knees and reaches forward to take the feet of the person in front of them, and place the feet on their belly.

> ** The bent knees create the points of the star.*

~ Now, each person reaches forward to place their hands on the waist of the person they face.

> ** This creates a deep arch in the back.*

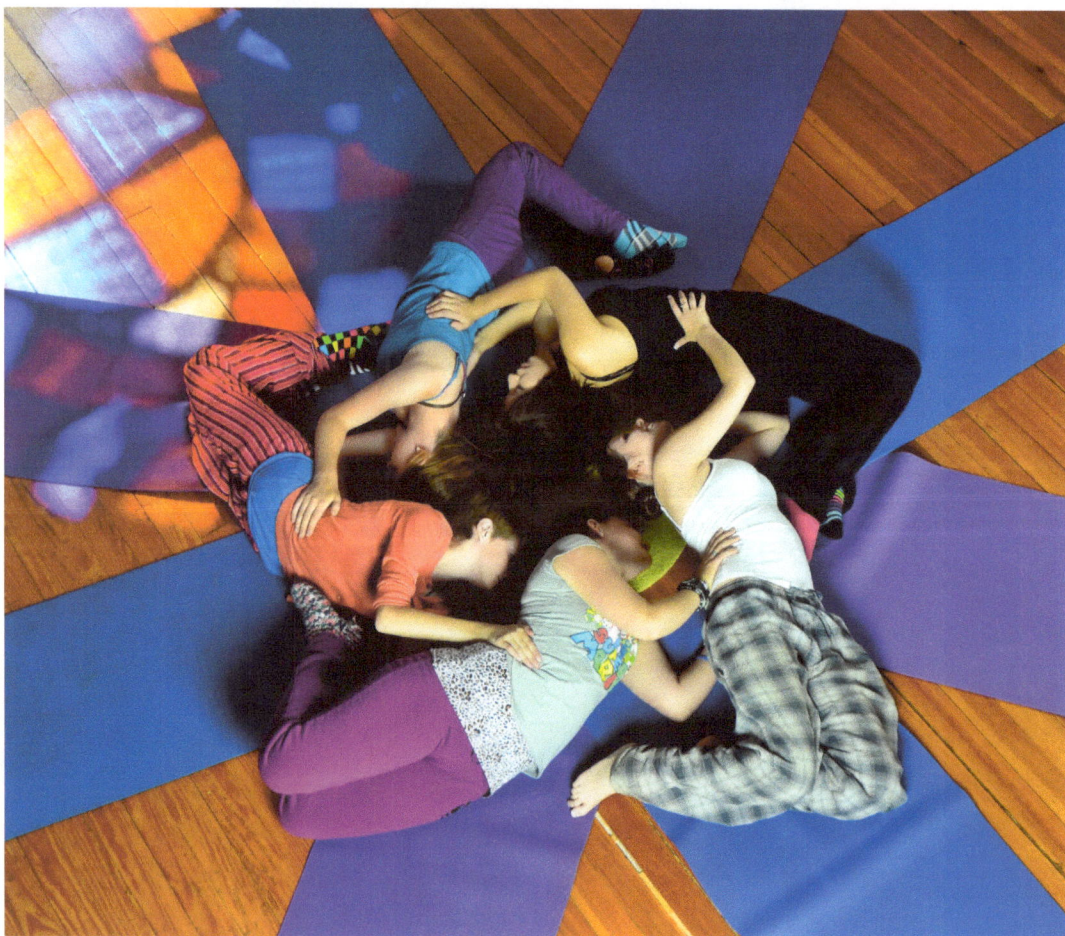

BINARY STAR

This pose requires four people.

MOVEMENT INSTRUCTIONS:

~ Begin with participants sitting back to back in Easy Sit Pose. Each person represents one of the four directions.

~ Participants place the left hand on the knee of the neighbor to their left, and the right hand on the knee of the neighbor to their right.

> ** Notice that participants' arms are now crossed over the arms of their neighbors.*

~ Each person pushes down gently into both hands, which helps to stretch each other's inner thigh muscles.

~ Participants seated in the North/South positions straighten their arms, open at a "T" and clasp hands with their partners.

~ People seated in the East/West positions do the same.

> ** Sit on the sitz bones with the spine straight and tall to feel the stretch in the pectoral muscles of the chest.*

> ** The top set of arms will be resting on the shoulders of the bottom set of arms. Make any adjustments you need to be comfortable*

> *Taller people should have the arms on top.*

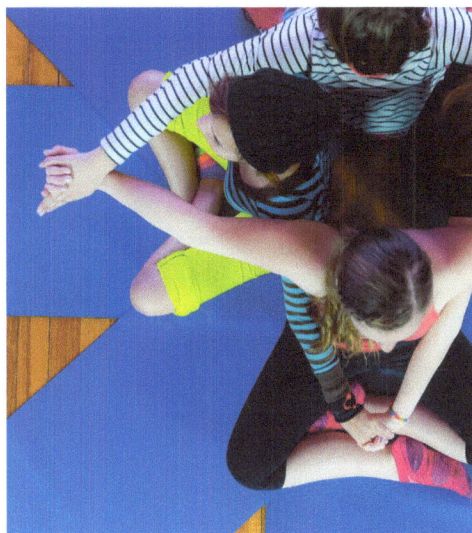

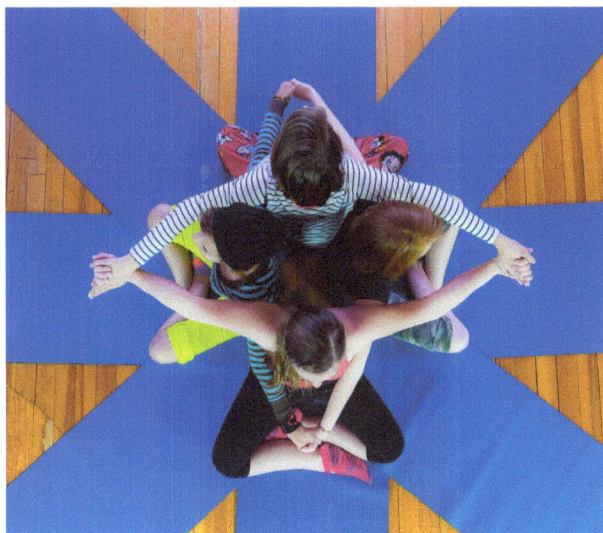

TURTLE FLOWER

This pose requires a minimum of six people but can be done with more.

MOVEMENT INSTRUCTIONS:

~ Begin by sitting in a circle with the legs in Butterfly Pose and your knees touching your neighbors' knees.

~ Lift the knees toward the center of the body, keeping the feet on the ground.

~ Bring the arms to the inside of the legs and thread them through the space underneath the knees.

~ Clasp hands with your neighbors on both sides.

~ Lean back, still holding hands, and lift the feet in the air. Find your balance.

~ Touch toes with your neighbors.

~ Alternate pointing and flexing your feet. When your feet are flexed toes will touch with your neighbors.

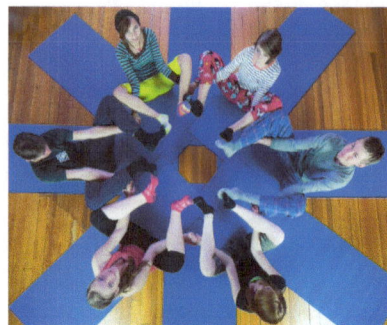

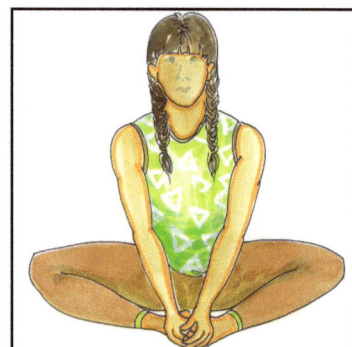

BUTTERFLY POSE

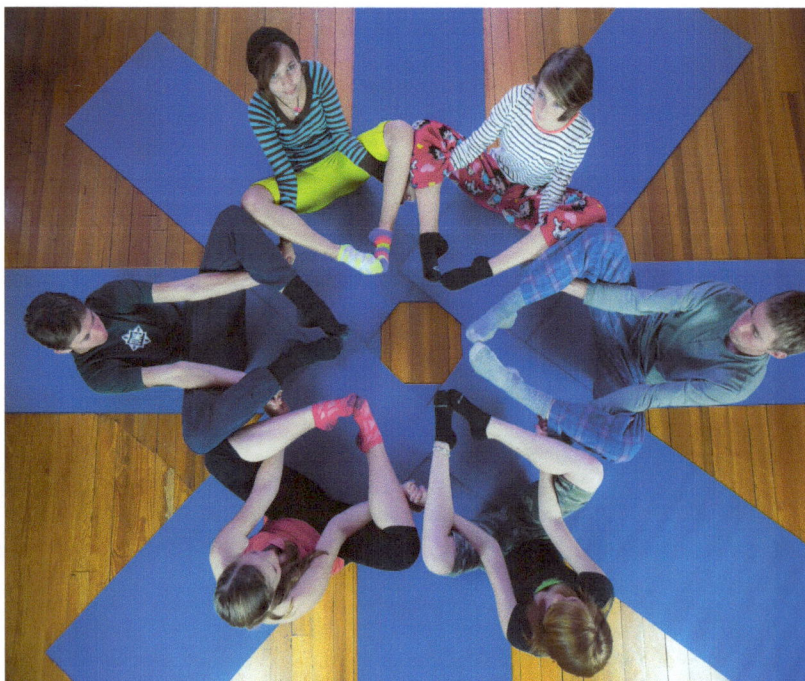

HUDDLE PUDDLE

This pose requires four people.

MOVEMENT INSTRUCTIONS:

~ Participants, each facing the center, sit with their legs in Butterfly Pose.

~ Lift into the crown of the head, with the chin parallel to the floor, and lengthen through the spine.

~ Each person slides his/her feet forward, toward the center of the circle, and opens the thighs into a diamond shape between the legs. Feel the stretch in the inner thigh muscles.

~ Bring your arms around the shoulders of your neighbors and gently lean forward. Allow the weight of your body, your neighbors' arms, and gravity to work as your torso slowly releases forward.

~ Drop the chin toward the chest to increase the stretch even more.

* This pose stretches the inner thigh muscles, the hamstrings, and the gluteal muscles.

* Coordinate the breath with other practitioners in the circle. This allows you to find a deeper release into the pose with each exhale.

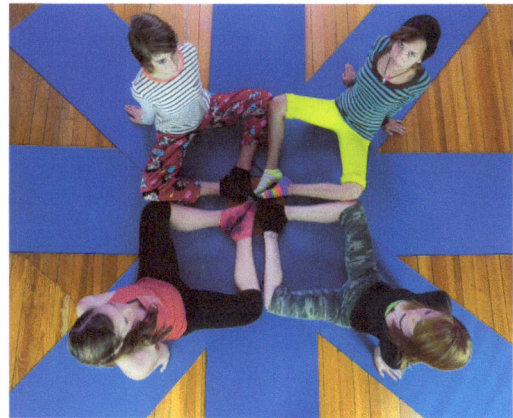

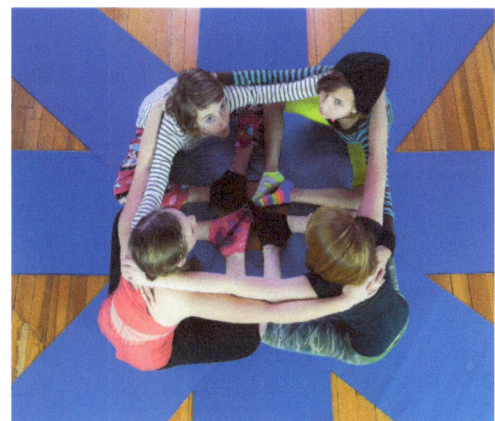

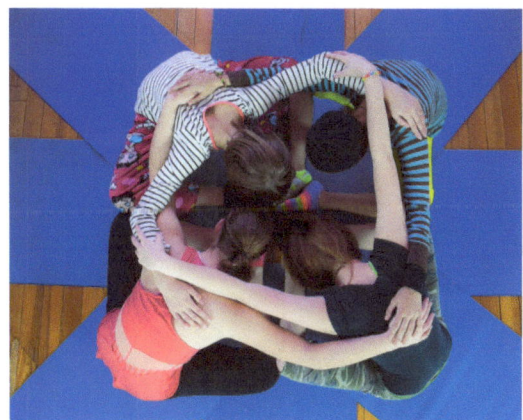

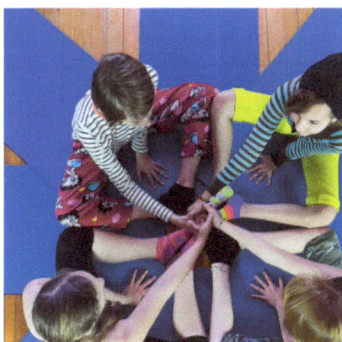

VARIATION

Instead of leaning in to achieve a stretch, participants can spiral the left hands together in the center to connect. Lean out reaching away with the right hand. This adds a nice stretch across the chest and arms.

~Be creative with hand options!

SUNFLOWER

This design shows requires eight people, but it can be done with any number of people.

MOVEMENT INSTRUCTIONS:

~ Practitioners sit in Staff Pose with the feet toward the center of the circle.

~ Point the toes toward the sky, straighten the spine, and rest the weight equally on both sitz bones. The crown of the head is lifted toward the sky.

~ Pull the toes back toward the nose and bring the hands to rest on the knees, or as far down the leg as your hamstrings can stretch while keeping the back straight.

~ Now, point the toes and slowly begin to lift the arms toward the sky.

~ As the arms rise, sink back and roll down the spine, one vertebra at a time, until you are lying on the floor. The toes are pointed and the fingers stretch in the opposite direction.

~ Take a deep breath and on the exhale, reverse the order of movement, using the abdominal muscles to slowly rise up into a seated position.

~ Reach for your toes!

> ** Perform the movement simultaneously with everyone in the circle. Synchronized movement creates the opening and closing of the flower petals.*
>
> ** Coordinate the movement with the breath: Inhale-arms come up. Exhale-spine rolls down.*
>
> ** Inhale-rest the body as you lie down. Exhale-use the breath to propel you back up to a seated position.*
>
> ** Each time you rise into a seated position, try to reach further down the leg to deepen the stretch in the hamstrings.*

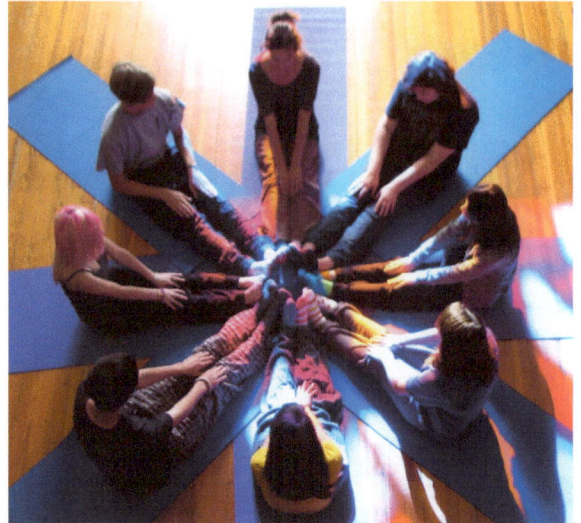

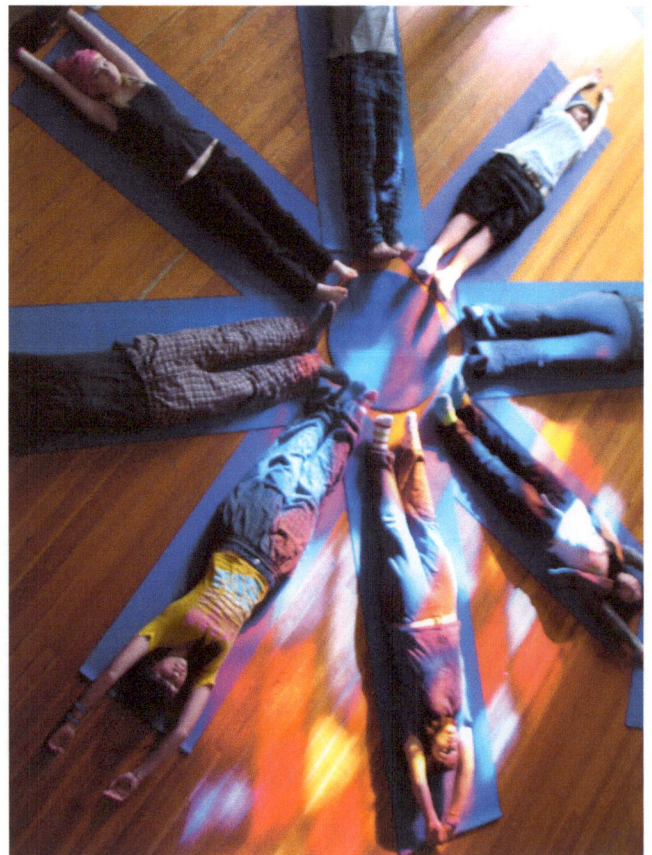

Snowflake

This design requires eight people.

Movement Instructions:

~ Begin by sitting together in a circle in Staff Pose.

~ Bend the legs so that the knees lift but the feet stay grounded.

~ Lean back to bring your weight onto the sitz bones as you lift the feet off of the ground. Keep the calves parallel to the floor.

~ Bring the arms out forward, alongside the legs and with the palms facing outwards.

> ** Use the abdominal muscles to maintain balance.*

~ Bring palms together with each of your neighbors to connect the circle.

~ Bring the arms up and, maintaining palm contact with your neighbors, rotate the arms around simultaneously. Use core strength to roll down the spine and straighten the legs.

> ** The final mandala is created when all practitioners are lying on their mats with their bodies straight and their arms open wide, connected to each other at the palms.*

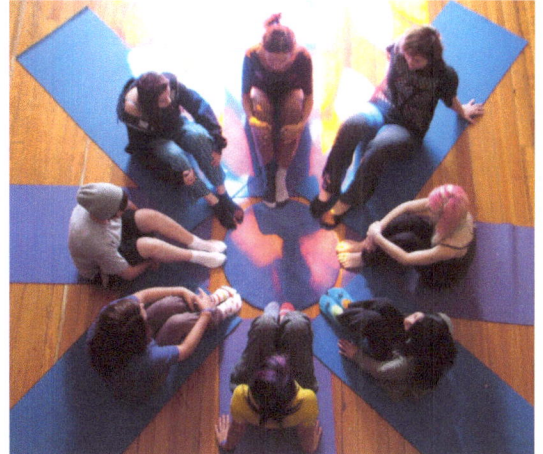

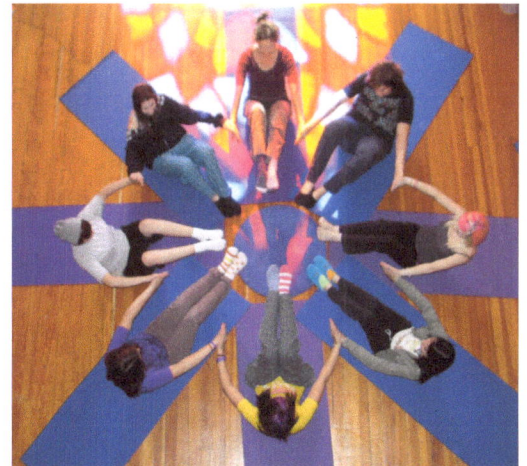

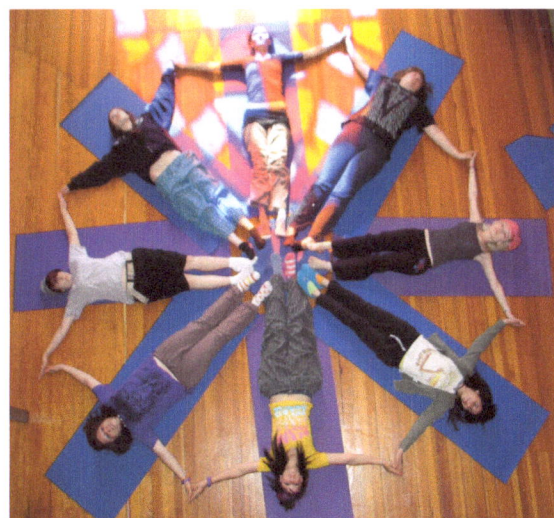

SNOWFLAKE LOOKS AND FEELS WONDERFUL WHEN ALL OF THE MOVEMENTS ARE SYNCHRONIZED!

WATER LILY

This requires eight people, divided into two teams of four. You can add in more pairs of two to create any design.

MOVEMENT INSTRUCTIONS:

~ Begin with four people sitting back to back in the four directions to create the inner circle. Each person sits with their legs straight and open wide. (Team 1)

~ Next, Team 2 sits facing Team 1 with their legs straight and wide open. The soles of the partners' feet touch, creating a diamond shape between each pair of people.

~ All practitioners sit up tall with the crowns of their heads lifted.

> ** Feel the stretch in the inner thigh muscles.*

~ Each pair, facing each other with the legs wide, extends their arms straight forward. Cross the arms at the elbows and clasp hands with your partner in the center of the diamond shape of the legs.

~ Now, both people gently pull forward by bending at the elbows.

> ** As the stretch increases, notice that you control the stretch by how much you pull forward.*

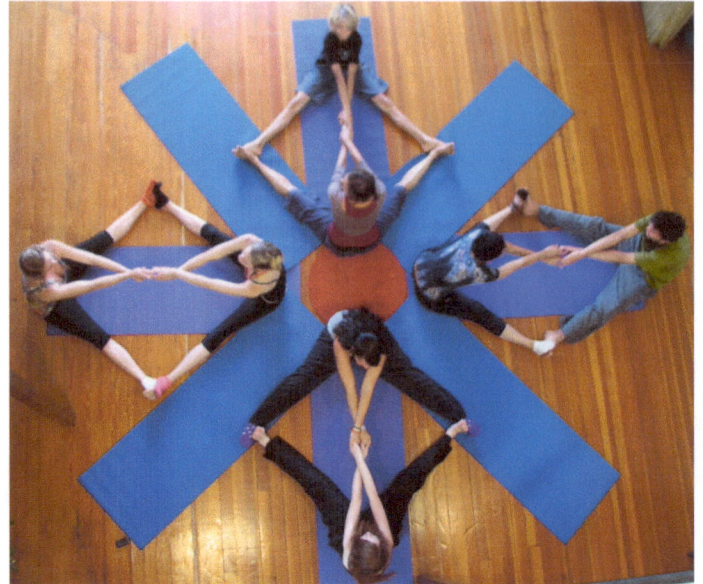

VARIATION

Turn to the person on the left or right and clasp hands with that person for a twist.

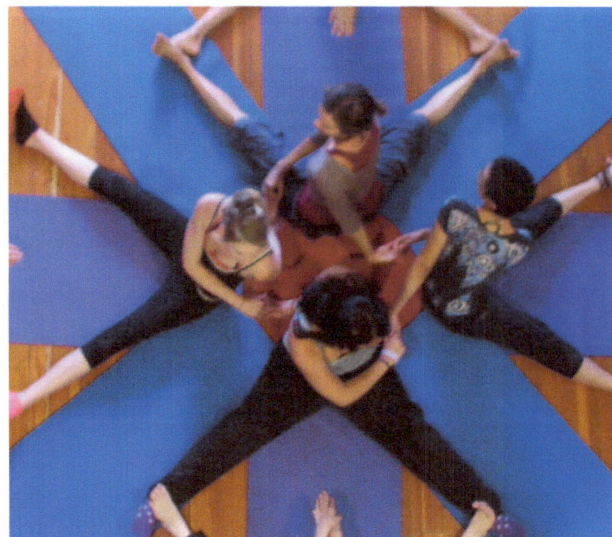

Star Fish

This pose can be done with six or eight people.

Star Fish is another pose that begins in the same configuration as Simple Flower, with the feet and head alternating toward the center.

Movement Instructions:

~ The four directions sit in Staff Pose while the midpoints lie in resting pose with their heads toward the center.

~ Each practitioner crosses the arms across the chest and clasps hands with the neighbors on either side.

This creates a square-shaped design with the arms.

With six people a triangle is made with the arms.

~ Once all hands are attached, practitioners who are seated in Staff Pose lean back gently to increase the stretch between the scapula.

* Be sure to communicate!*

* This is an excellent stretch for the space between the shoulder blades.*

* Take deep breaths into the back of the ribs.*

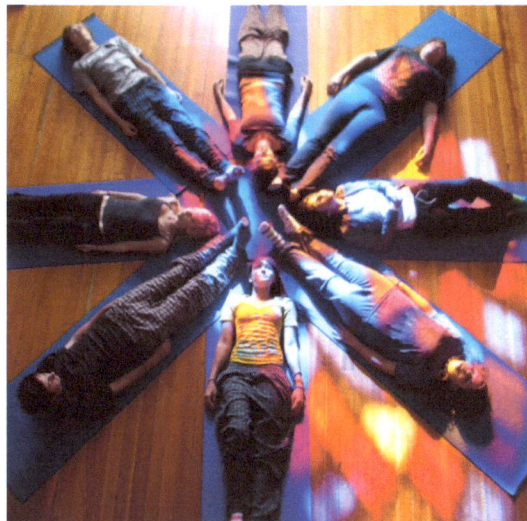

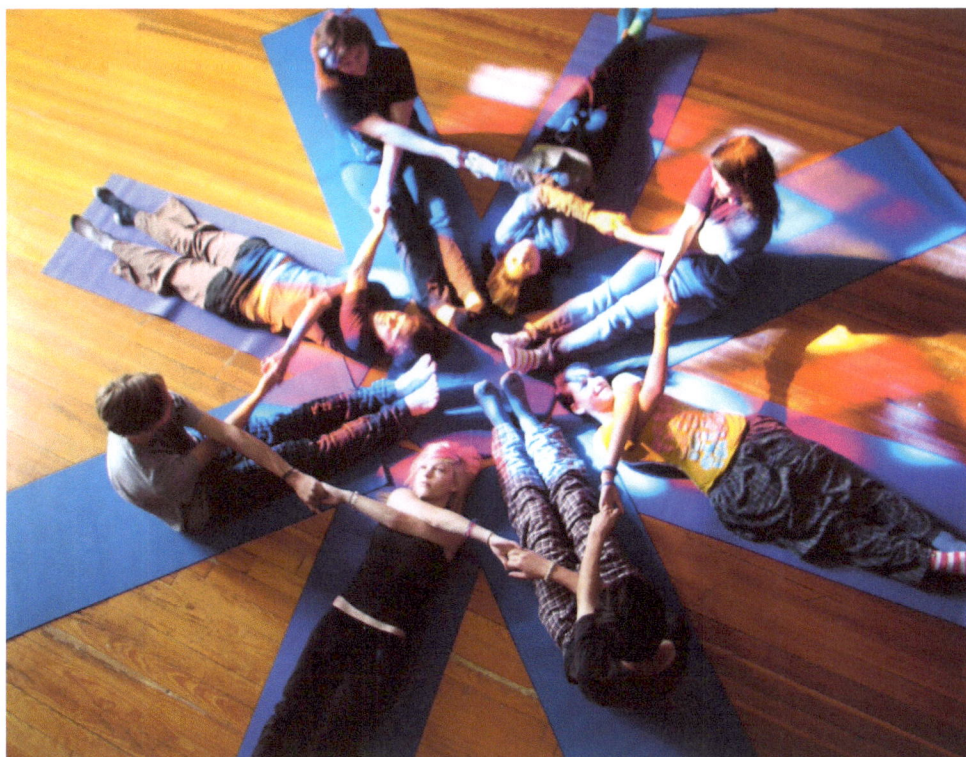

CIRCLE OF FALLEN TREES

This pose requires six people, who create the design one person at a time.

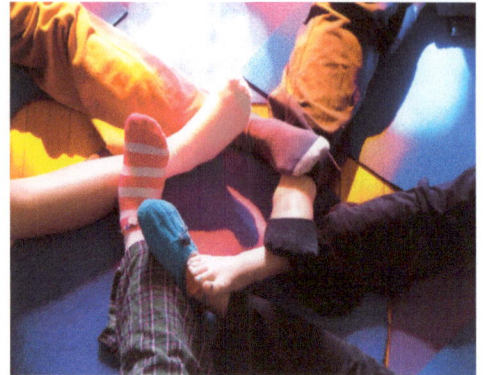

MOVEMENT INSTRUCTIONS:

~ The first practitioner is seated with his/her right leg straightened and resting on the ground.

> ** At this point, there is no center. The center becomes clear as each person places his/her foot.*

~ The second person now places the arch of the right foot to touch the ankle of the first person. Then, the third person places the arch of the right foot to touch the ankle of the second person, and so on until all six people have placed their foot. This creates the inner circle design.

~ All practitioners lie down onto their backs.

> ** The right legs are all straight and resting on the ground, while the left legs are bent with the knees facing the sky and the left feet on the ground.*

~ Next, bring the arms up straight upward, reaching toward the sky.

~ Each person straightens their bent leg and places their heel into the outstretched hands of the person to the left of them. This creates the full expression of the pose.

> ** Everyone should be balanced and supporting each other comfortably.*

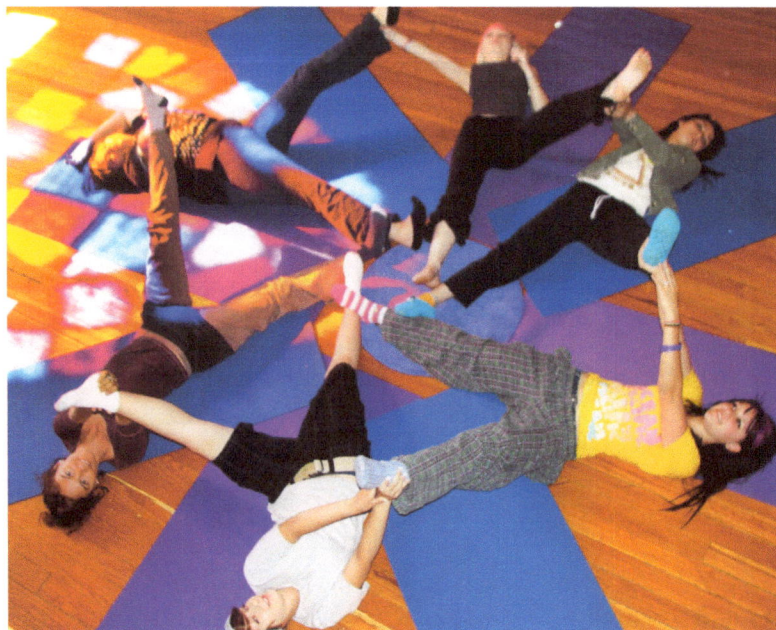

CORKSCREW

This pose requires six to ten people.

~ Begin with practitioners seated and facing the center of the circle with their knees bent and their feet on the ground, a little more than hip-distance apart.

~ Bring both knees down to the left side to initiate a gentle twist in the torso.

~ Supporting the body with the left hand, bring the right arm up and around, placing the right hand on the floor parallel with the left hand.

~ Feel the twist deepen in the torso.

* Make sure your shoulders are parallel to each other.

* The arms should be straight lines from the wrists to the shoulders.

* Mind your breath: Inhale to lengthen up through the crown of the head and exhale to twist a little deeper.

~ Bring the right hand back up and around the body and then down to support as you slowly unwind the torso to exit the pose.

~ The knees come up to the center. Gently rock the knees back and forth to release and integrate the stretch.

~ Begin the same movements to the opposite side, allowing the knees to move down toward the right.

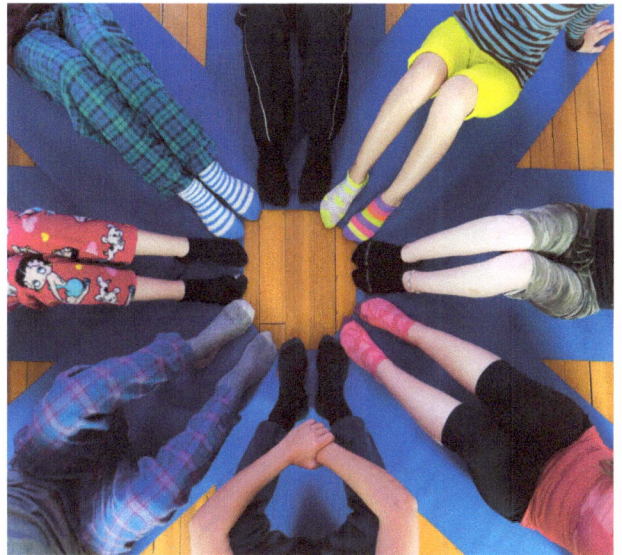

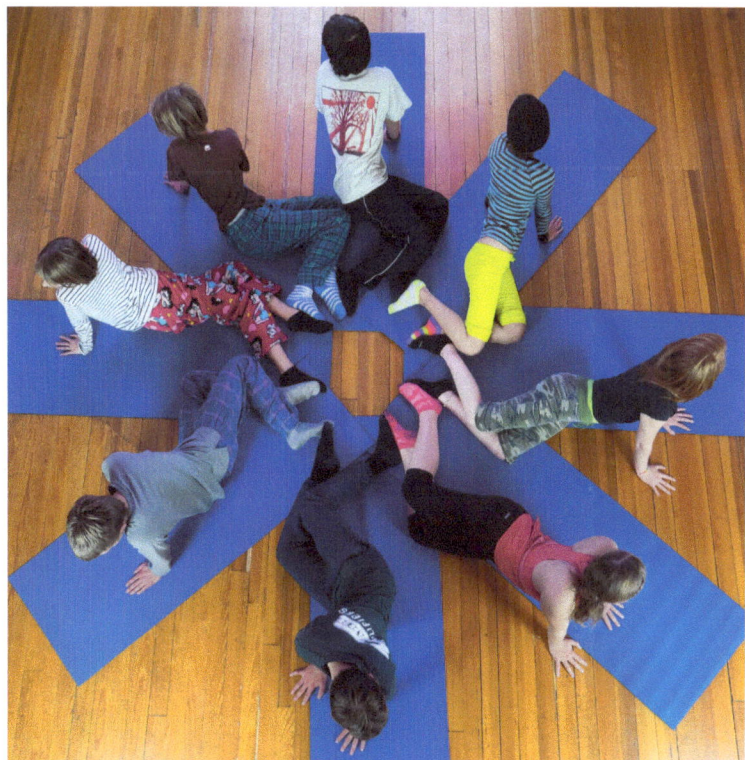

35

WINE OPENER:
VARIATION OF THE CORKSCREW

This pose requires eight people.

MOVEMENT INSTRUCTIONS:

~ From Corkscrew, walk the hands forward and rest the entire front of the torso down on the floor.

~ Rest the head on the floor, facing the direction of the knees.

> ** This is a gentle, supported spinal twist. Be sure to make any adjustments so that you are comfortable.*

~ Extend the top leg straight toward the center of the circle and allow it to hover above the ground.

~ Slowly allow the foot lower to touch the floor.

~ Bring the arms into a T-position and connect hands with your neighbors to create the outside circumference of the circle.

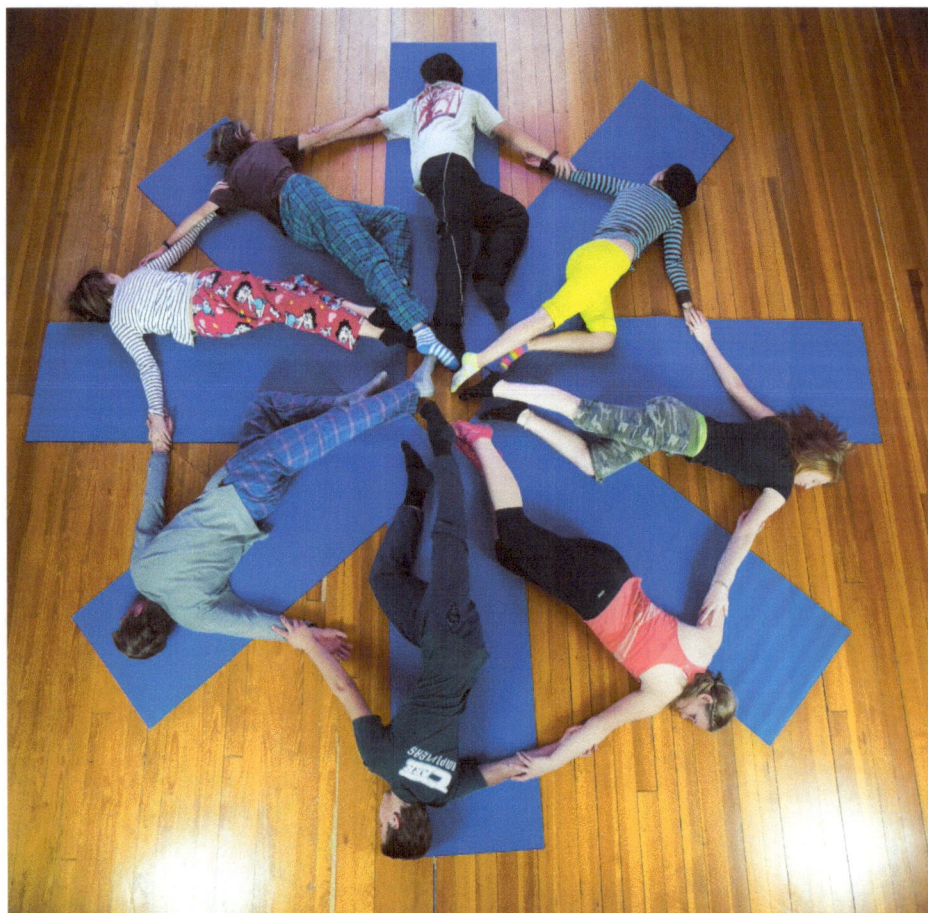

Four Leaf Clover

This pose requires four people.

Movement Instructions:

~ Each practitioner bends the left leg at the knee so that the knee points in toward the center of the circle.

> ** The heel of the left foot will rest by the right hip.*

~ Wrap the right leg over the left and bend the right leg at the knee so that both knees line up with one another.

> ** The heel of the right foot will rest by the left hip.*

> ** Stacking the knees takes a great deal of flexibility. You may have to work up to this strong stretch by bringing the ankle onto the thigh near the knee and incrementally move the ankle forward as your muscles allow.*

~ Flex the feet and touch toes with your neighbors to create the circumference of the circle.

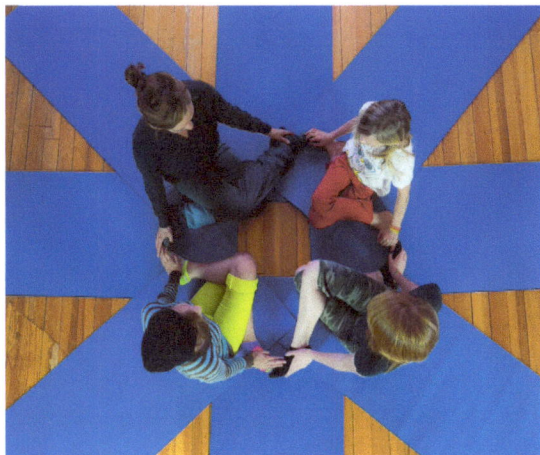

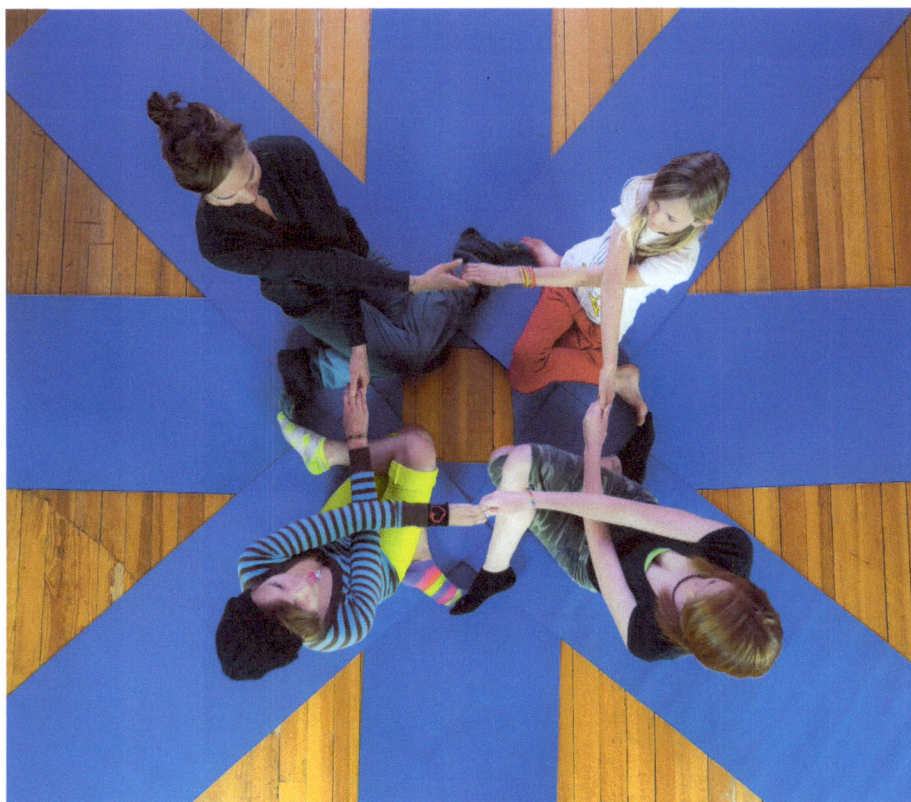

~ There are many things that you can do with the arms to have fun with the design, such as:

~ Cuddle (arms on the shoulders)

~ Hand spiral

~ Lean back

~ Cross hands

Get creative and see what designs you can make!

Sea Anemone

This pose can be done with any number of people.

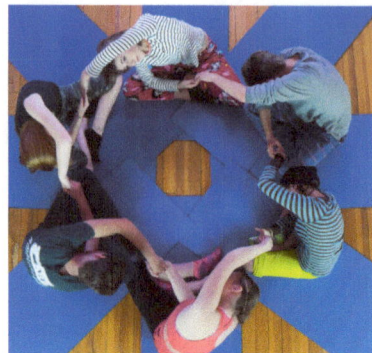

Movement Instructions:

~ Begin by sitting in a circle in Easy Sit Pose, resting the palms of the hands on the knees.

> * The knees of each person should lightly touch his/her neighbors' knees at the edges.

~ Inhale deeply and as you exhale, drop into the sitz bones and lift into the crown of the head. Feel the spine extend and lengthen.

~ All practitioners inhale the left arm up and overhead, bending at the torso and bringing the hand over toward the right side of the body.

~ Simultaneously, curl the right arm under and across the midline to the left, allowing the back of the palm to rest on the left knee.

> * Everyone is poised to connect hands.

~ Each person connects the upper left hand with the lower right hand of the person to their right.

~ Take several deep breaths here.

> * Feel the side of the body extend and open.

> * Be sure to keep the sitz bones anchored to the ground.

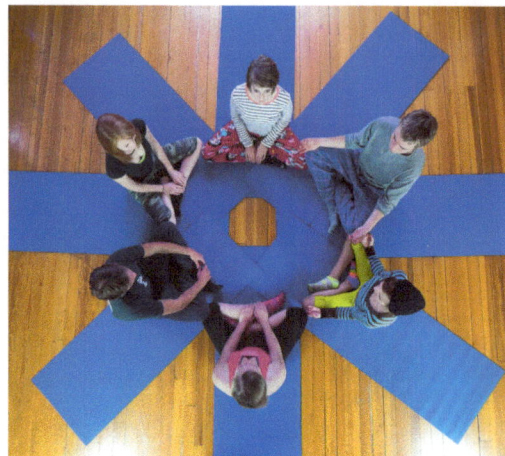

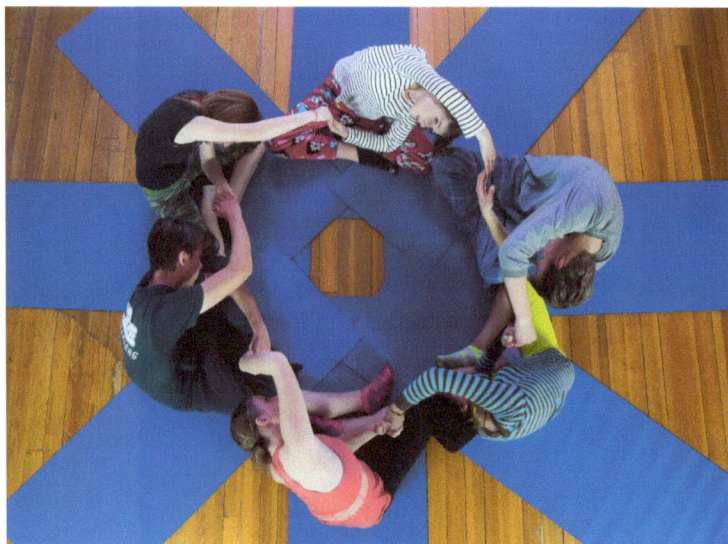

~ Come out of the stretch slowly, then repeat on the other side.

NAUTILUS

This pose can be done with four or more people.

MOVEMENT INSTRUCTIONS:

~ Begin with all practitioners arranged in a circle and seated.

~ Turn slightly to the right, so that each person's left knee points in toward the center of the circle.

~ Reach forward with the left hand and back with the right hand.

~ Connect hands with both of your neighbors.

> ** The forward left hand will connect with the back right hand of the person in front.*

> ** The elbows are gently bent and the body should be comfortable. Make any adjustments before moving forward.*

~ Inhale deeply and as you exhale, straighten the arms and lift into the crown of the head.

> ** Make sure the sitz bones are anchored evenly to the floor.*

> ** Feel the spine twist up the entire torso.*

> ** Try to square the shoulders and create a lift in the chest, as if you are lifting the heart.*

~ Slowly release and repeat to the other side.

> ** Do not forget to switch the legs in Easy Sit Pose, bringing the opposite leg to the front.*

Keep the elbows bent. Simultaneously, lean the heads in toward the center of the circle. Keep the sitz bones anchored as you rotate the chest and gaze up toward the sky.

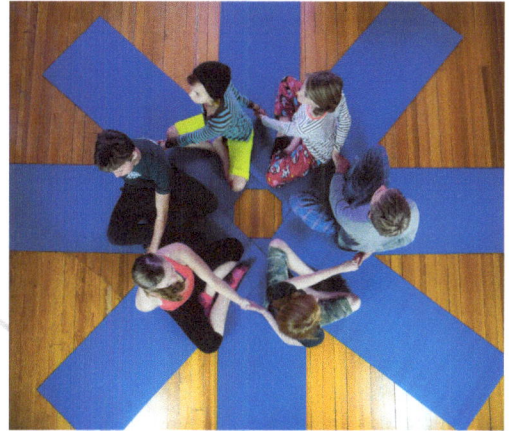

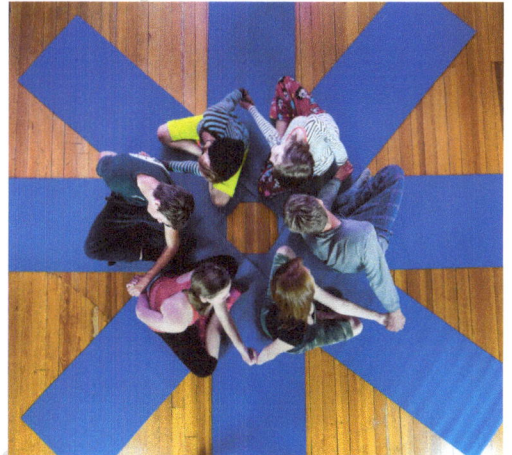

HAND SPIRAL

This pose can be done with four or more people.

MOVEMENT INSTRUCTIONS:

~ Participants bring left hands to toward the center with the thumbs facing up towards the sky and fingertips touching.
~ Curl the finger tips in and watch the spiral emerge in the hands.

~Place the thumbs down along the outer edge or circumference of the spiral.

~ Now, all participants lean away from the center and reach extend the right arm out at a T.

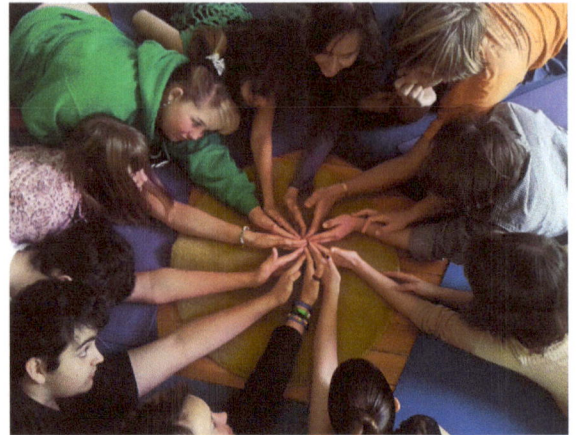

PREPERATION FOR HAND SPIRAL

Once you have mastered the Spiral 1, you can take it further by adding a second Spiral with the right hands.

DOUBLE SPIRAL (NOT PICTURED)

This pose can be done with four or more people.

MOVEMENT INSTRUCTIONS:

~ Bring the right hands to connect above the left hands.

~ Now spiral in toward the center.

~Find a secure grip in both spirals and lean back, arms extended.

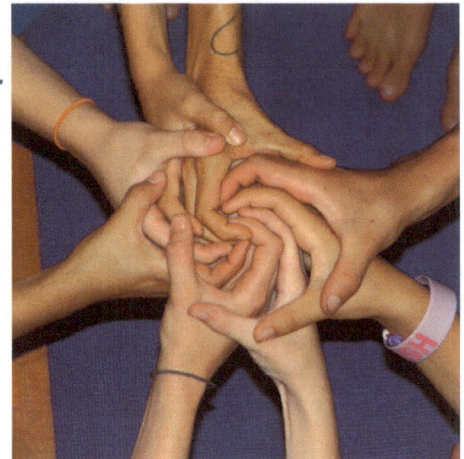

HAND SPIRAL

Feel the stretch along the outer arms and into the shoulders and shoulder blades.

Breathe Deep.

DOUBLE REVERSE SPIRAL

This pose can be done with four or more people.

MOVEMENT INSTRUCTIONS:

~Do a Hand Spiral with the left hands, thumbs face up.

~Now bring the right hands in toward the center above the left hands, with the thumbs face down! Spiral in towards the center to find a secure grip. Lift the right hands to the sky while dropping the left hands toward the ground.

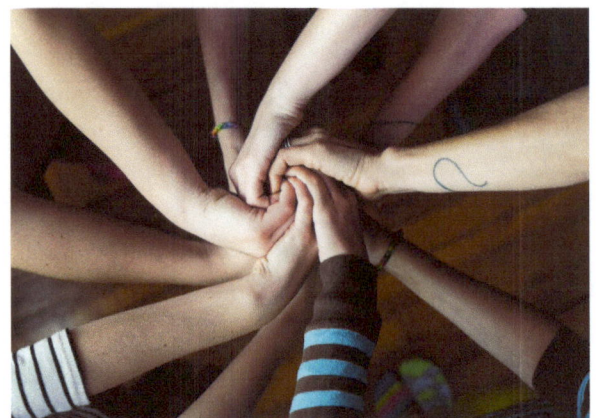

DOUBLE REVERSE SPIRAL

Hand Star

This pose can be done with four or more people.

Movement Instructions:

~All participants bring hands to the center palms face down.

~Turn the hands to the side (thumb facing the sky) and bring the tips of the fingers toward the center.

~Bend the fingers, curling them into a hand spiral.

~Lift the index finger and the thumb.

~Connect every other thumb and index finger together, weaving them together to make the star design.

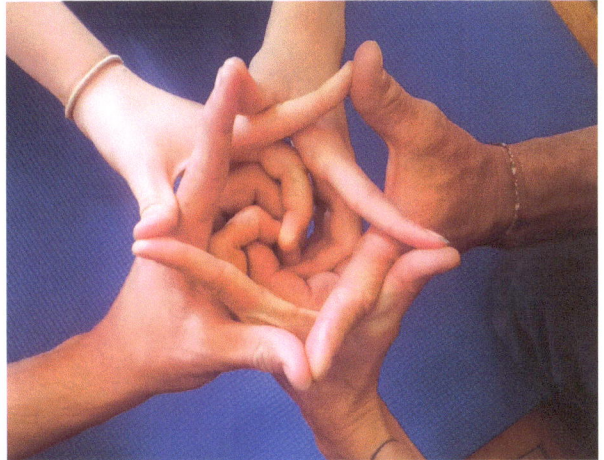

HAND STAR

Thumb Ring (Cosmic Hitchhiker)

This pose can be done with four or more people.

Movement Instructions:

~ All participants bring the right hands forward with the thumbs facing up (like a hitchhiker).

~ Turn the thumbs to the left and connect, each hand holding each thumb to form a solid ring.

* Try a Double Thumb Ring by connecting with the thumbs on the left hands also.

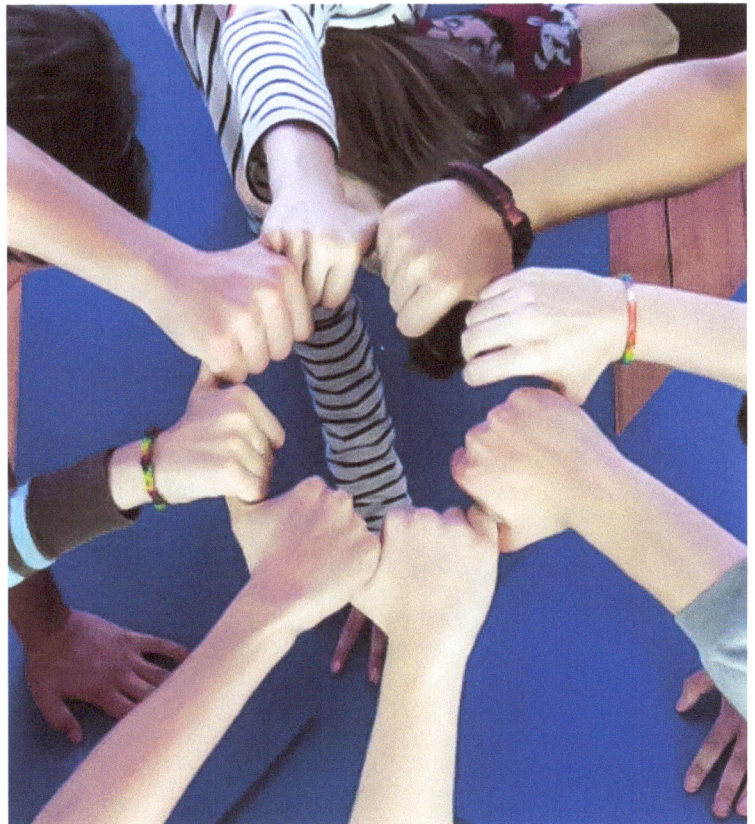

POPCORN TWIST

This pose can be done with four or more people.

MOVEMENT INSTRUCTIONS:

~ Begin by standing in a circle, each practitioner facing the center.

~ Cross the arms in front of the body, beginning with the left arm over the right. It is important that everyone has the same arm on top.

~ All participants connect hands with your neighbors.

~ Stand, facing toward the center, with the left arm over the right, and the hands joined with your neighbors. Simultaneously, open the left arm up and over the head, which twists the body around to the left.

~ When the movement is executed properly, everyone faces outward instead of in toward the center of the circle.

~ Now facing out, fold forward, releasing the head down towards the floor.

~Slowly roll back up one vertebra at a time.

~ Practice reversing the movement so that you finish in the original position, facing forward.

> ** Once the group has practiced and understands the twist, the movement can be created in an instant with a jump!*
>
> ** This pose is great for increasing range of motion in the shoulders.*
>
> ** Begin with just four people to keep it simple, but add more once the group understands the motion.*
>
> ** This pose takes some practice but it is fun! Popcorn Twist is excellent for fostering teamwork.*

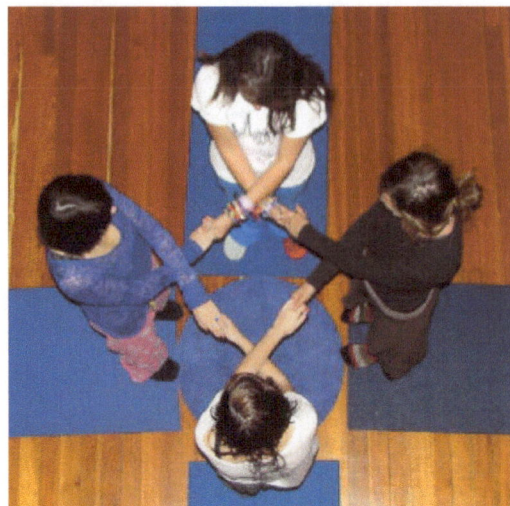

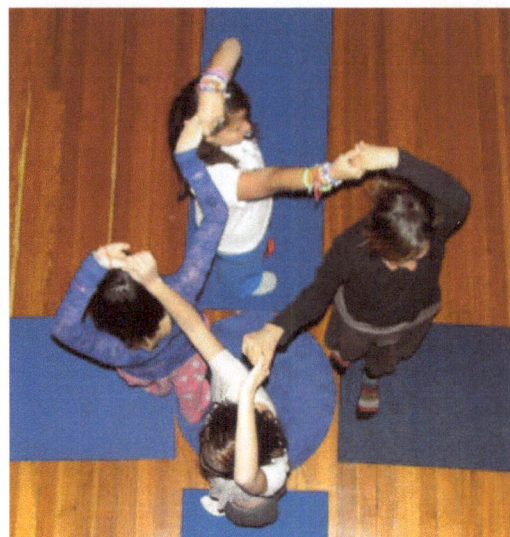

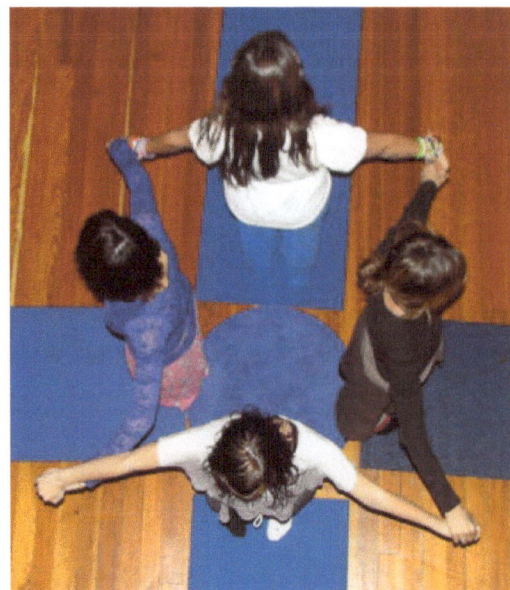

FLOWER OF LIFE

This pose requires six people divided into two teams of three.

MOVEMENT INSTRUCTIONS:

~Begin with three people (Team 1) sit down, facing away from each other with legs in a wide Butterfly Pose.

~ The other three people (Team 2) sit down opening their legs into a wide straddle, forming a triangle around Team 1.

~ Team 2 connects hands behind the back of Team 1.

> * This is a deep stretch for the inner thigh muscles.

> * When group one connects hands, it not only increases their inner thigh stretch, but it also increases the stretch for Team 2 (in Butterfly Pose).

> * Come out of the pose slowly. Then, switch teams so that both groups can experience the different sensations caused by the alternative stretch.

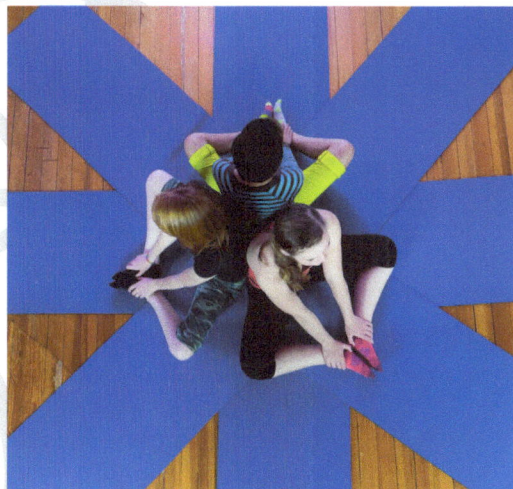

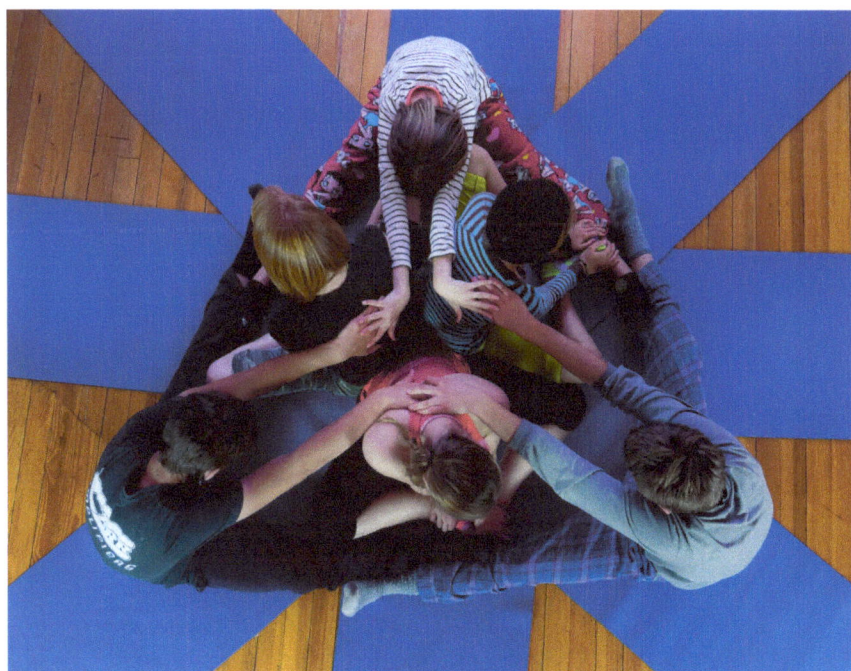

DANDELION
This pose requires eight to ten people.

MOVEMENT INSTRUCTIONS:

~ Begin with eight people lying on their bellies with their heads toward the center of the circle.

~ Bring the arms forward in long straight lines and place the hands palm to palm, in prayer position. This creates a center flower design with the arms.

~ Aim the head forward and place the chin on the floor as you cast your gaze toward your hands.

~ Bring the legs into long straight lines, placing the tops of the feet against the floor.

~ Gently push the pubic bone toward the floor to stabilize the body. Then, begin to extend into the legs and arms simultaneously. This stretches the entire front body.

~ Relax the body, place your head to the side, and take several breaths.

~ Bring the head to center once again, this time resting the forehead on the floor.

~Open the legs wide enough to touch feet with both neighbors. Push into the pubic bone and tighten the muscles in the legs as you extend the feet and hands in opposite directions.

~ After several breaths, relax and let the muscles go limp.

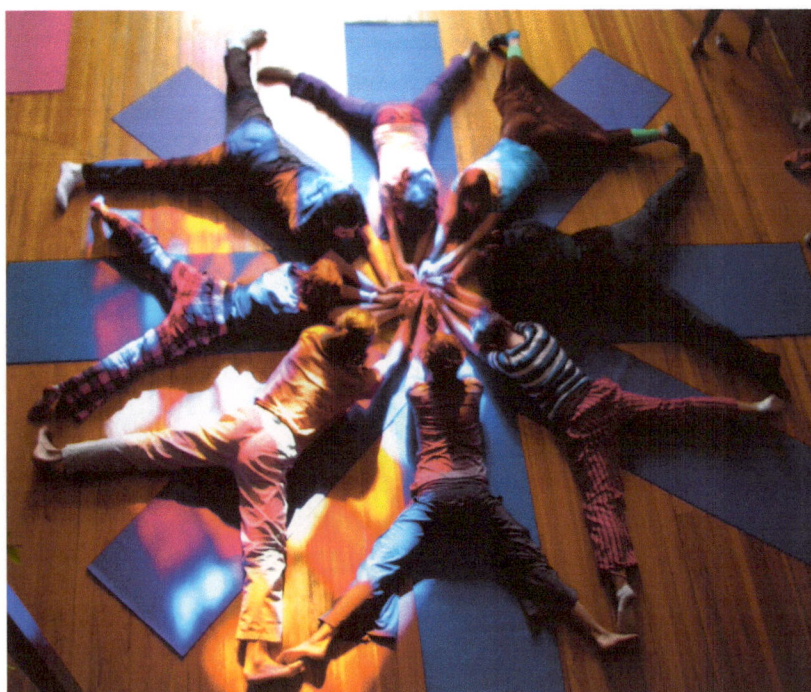

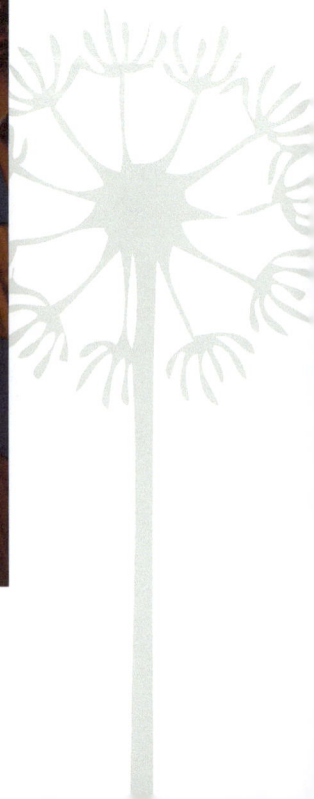

DANDELION (CONTINUED)

The final stage of this pose is only to be done if the body feels comfortable with a strong arch in the back. It may take some time to work up to this.

~ All practitioners place their heads to one side (the same side for everyone) and bring the arms back along side the body.

~ Bend the legs at the knees.

~ Each person clasps the ankles of both neighbors.

~ Once the hands and ankles are connected throughout the circle, everyone simultaneously rolls the shoulders up and away from the floor.

~ If it feels comfortable, try to reach the feet up toward the sky.

Do not rock forward or backward.

Keep the arms straight.

~ Release the ankles and bring the arched spine down slowly.

Come into Child's Pose to rest and counterbalance the back.

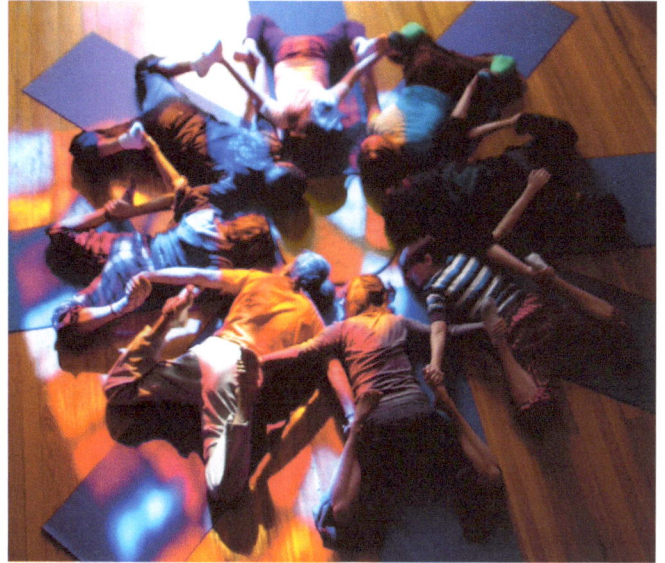

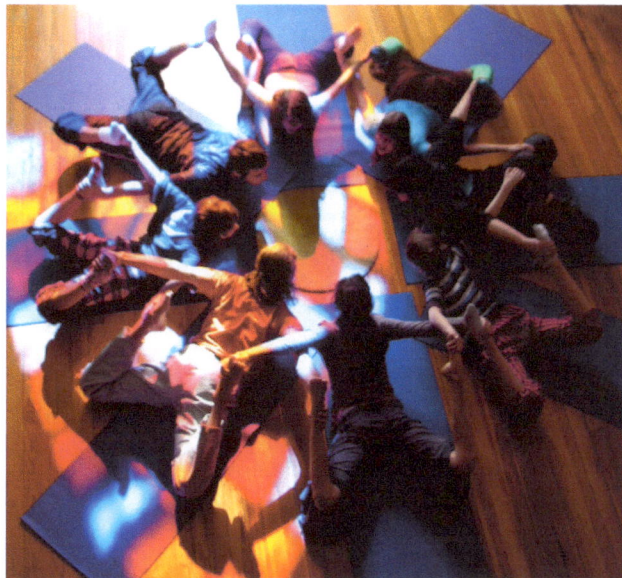

This pose stretches and strengthens the chest, shoulders, abdominal muscles, thighs and back!

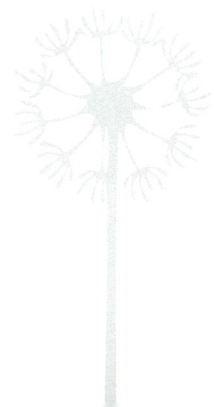

FRACTAL

This pose requires eight people divided into two teams of four.

MOVEMENT INSTRUCTIONS:

~ Begin with four people, Team 1 seated in Butterfly Pose and facing the center.

~ Slide the legs forward to create a diamond shape between the legs.

~ The feet of all practitioners should meet in the center to create a four leaf clover.

~ The practitioners in Team 2 sit behind each person in Team 1, who also face the center of the circle.

~ Practitioners in Team 2 wrap their legs around their Team 1 partner, bringing the soles of the feet together in front the person in Team 1.

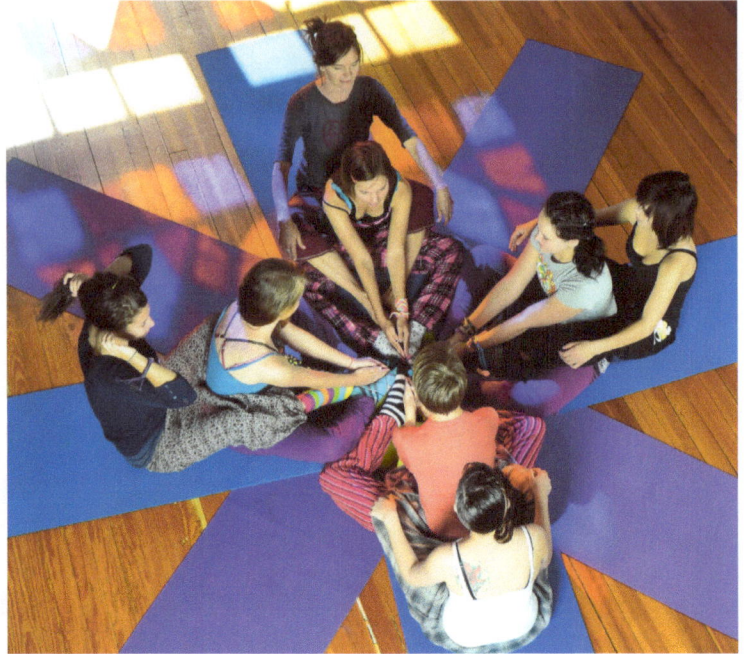

* Both team members' feet are inside the diamond space in between both sets of legs.

* The extra weight of the second pair of legs on top of the butterfly will increase the inner thigh stretch for Team 1.

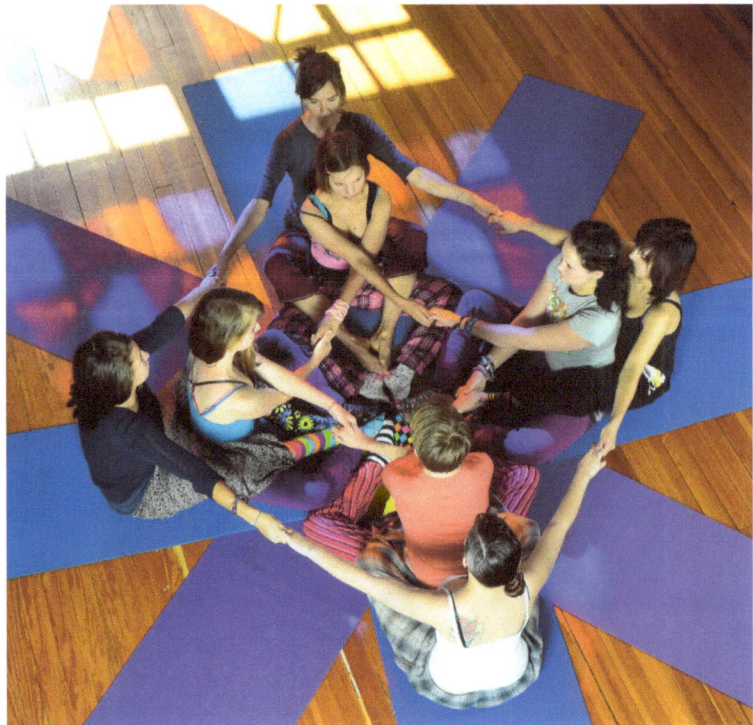

FRACTAL (CONTINUED)

~ Practitioners in Team 2 lie down on their backs, their legs still wrapped around Team 1 members and the soles of their feet together.

~ Team 2 opens the arms out wide into a T-shape with the palms facing toward the sky.

~ Team 1 also opens their arms out wide to a T and lies back on top of the practitioners in Team 2.

~ Team 1 places the backs of their hands in the open palms of Team 2.

~ Rest and breathe here. Then slowly exit the pose and switch groups to repeat.

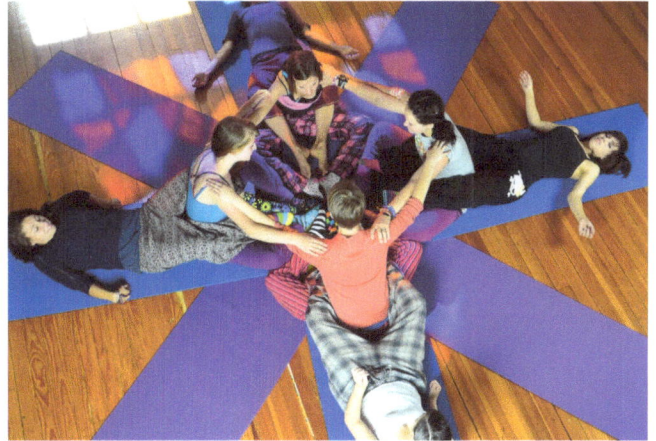

* Both groups may need to bend the arms at the elbows in order to place the hands together.

* This pose stretches the muscles of the chest and the inner thighs.

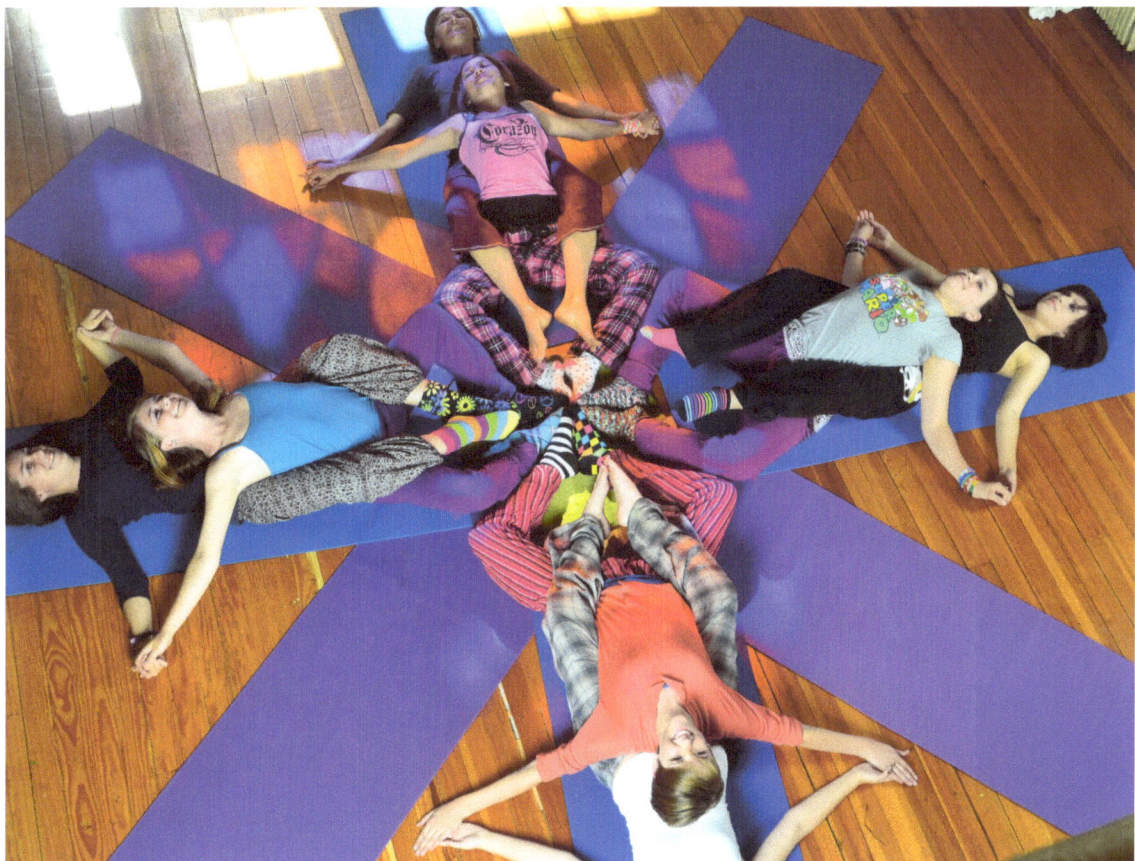

SUNSHINE

This pose can be done with six or more people.

MOVEMENT INSTRUCTIONS:

~ Begin with a group of people lying on their bellies, heads toward the center of the circle.

~ Each person crisscrosses the arms by bringing the left arm across the middle of the body (toward the right) and the right arm across the middle of the body (toward the left).

> ** The arms cross at the center of the chest, which stretches in between the scapula.*

~ Everyone connects hands with their neighbors.

~ Lift into the crown of the head, keeping the nose pointing toward the center.

~ Straighten out through the legs and press down into the pubic bone to stabilize the back.

~ Tuck the toes and push into the ball of the feet.

~ Energize through the legs by lifting the knees off the ground and pulling the kneecaps up toward the pelvis.

~ Release the pose and rest for a moment.

~ Reverse the arms so that the opposite arm is on top and repeat the actions of the pose.

> ** Deep breaths increase the stretch in the rhomboid muscles between the scapula.*

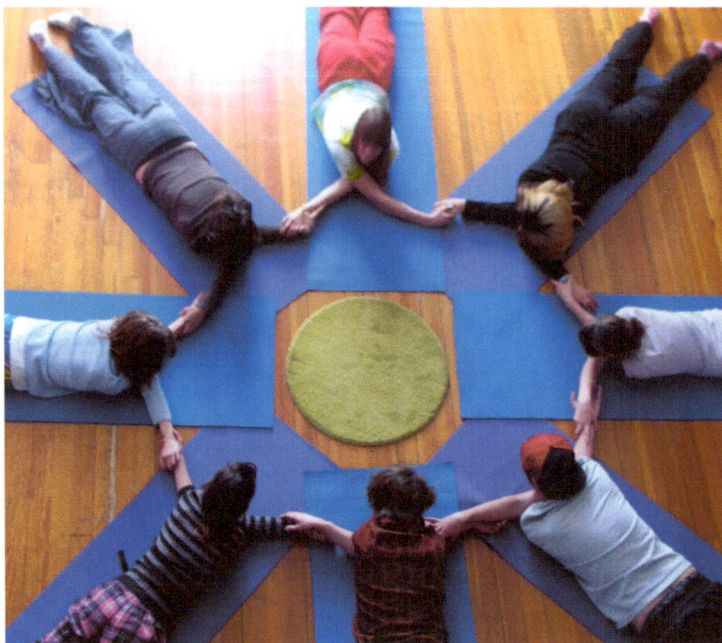

WHIRLIE BIRD

This pose requires eight people divided into two teams of four.

MOVEMENT INSTRUCTIONS:

~ Begin with four people, Team 1 sitting back to back, the legs open in a wide straddle.

~ Practitioners in Team 2, also in a wide-legged straddle, sit across from and facing Team 1.

~ The feet of Team 1 meet up with the feet of Team 2. The partners on each team join right hands.

~ Inhale as you lengthen the spine and on the exhale, reach the left hand over toward the right and clasp hands with your neighbor at a diagonal line.

* This is a deep stretch for the whole side body and the inner thigh muscles, which should be attempted only if it feels comfortable.

~ Release and bring your position back to neutral before you begin this movement on the opposite side.

~ Partners connect left hands as they lift into the crown of the head and lengthen the spine.

~ With the right hand, reach across at a diagonal toward the left to connect hands with your neighbor.

~ Exit the pose slowly and take several deep breaths. Then, connect both hands with the person directly across from you. Inhale as you lift into the crown of the head and exhale as you drop the shoulders down the back and away from the ears.

Modifications: Bend the knees.

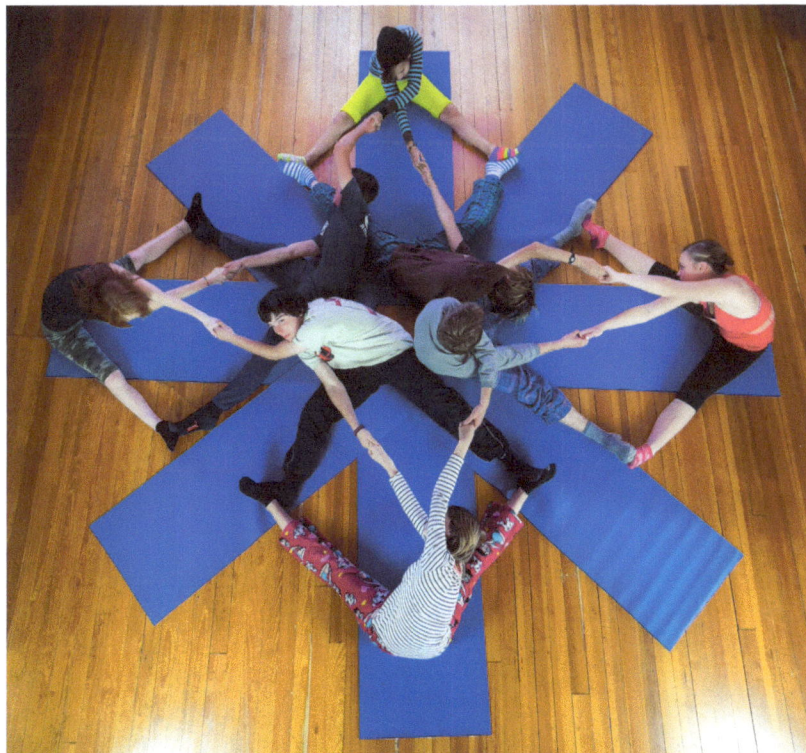

LOTUS FLOWER

This pose requires eight people divided into two teams of four.

MOVEMENT INSTRUCTIONS:

~ Team 1: Begin with the inner circle of four people sitting in the four directions. North/South are back to back, as is East/West. All participants sit facing the outside of the circle.

> ** This leaves a small square at the very center of the mandala.*

~ Team 1 opens their legs wide and bends their knees slightly.

~ Team 2 places themselves at the midpoints in between each person in Team 1 and sits facing toward the center of the circle with legs open wide and a slight bend at the knees.

~ Participants in Team 2 connect one hand and one foot with the two people from Team 1 that create the directional corner (SW, SE, NW, NE).

> ** Notice that the connection is with only one foot and one hand.*

> ** The balls of the feet are connected, while the heels rest on the ground with knees still bent.*

~ Team 2 leans back, shifting slightly onto the tailbone, and gets ready to lift the legs.

> ** The next movement is a collective movement where everyone must work together.*

~ In unison, both teams gently push into the feet, lifting the heels off the ground until the feet are sole to sole and the shins form one long line from knee to knee.

~ Breathe and balance! If you want to take the pose further, you can try to straighten the legs and create a V-shape.

~ This is a full expression of the challenging lotus flower mandala. To create this pose, all participants must work together. It takes practice! If at first you don't succeed, try again.

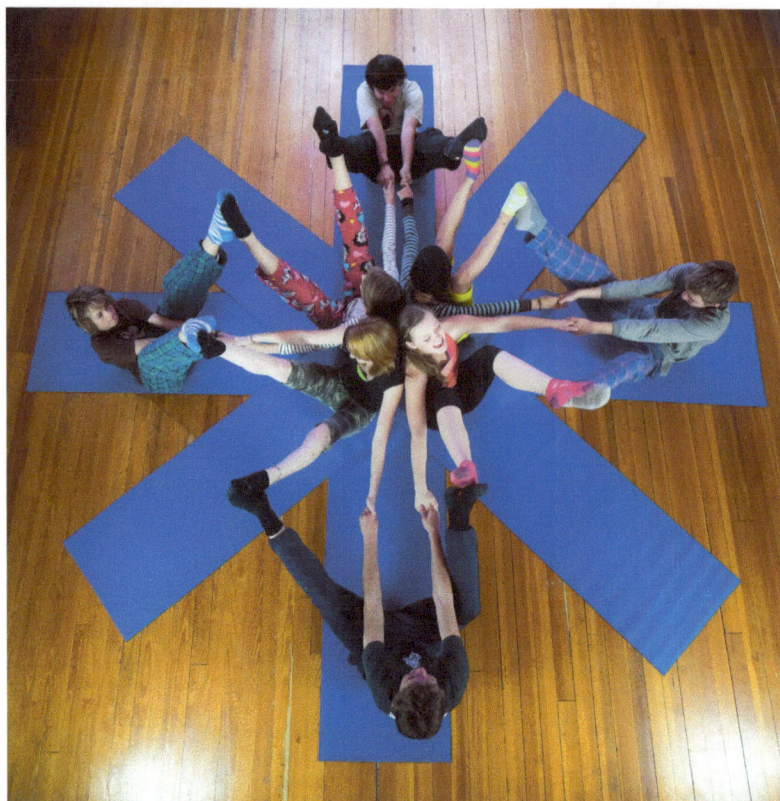

DOUBLE DECKER

This pose requires eight people, divided into two teams of four.

MOVEMENT INSTRUCTIONS:

> ** It is important that the participants are of similar weight and height. The heavier people should be positioned as the "tables."*

~ The first group of four practitioners assume Table Position, on their hands and knees with their heads facing the center.

~ The next group of four (the "planks") stand on the right side of each table.

~ Each plank slowly lies down with his/her face toward the floor, lengthwise on top of the backs of the tables.

> ** The planks place their lower bellies on the lower back of the tables.*

~ The planks use their arms to support their upper body weight, as if one is doing a push up.

Special Directions for Planks:

> ** Make sure your arms are straight with the elbow over the wrists. Proper alignment is important to give the pose integrity.*
>
> ** Stay strong! Do not sag in the shoulders and keep the back aligned from neck to tailbone. This creates strong core muscles.*

Special Directions for Tables:

> ** Make sure your back is flat like a table. Do not sag in the back or shoulders and keep your core muscles engaged.*

~ Each plank rests his/her feet on the upper back of the previous plank.

> ** The top deck is now woven together, perfectly balanced and supported. Breathe and enjoy the pose!*

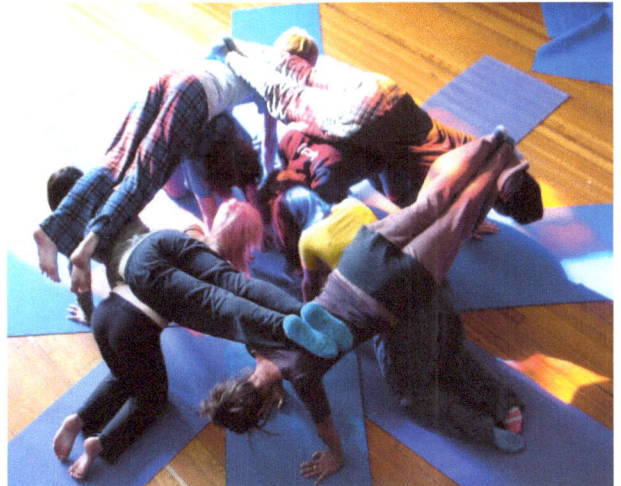

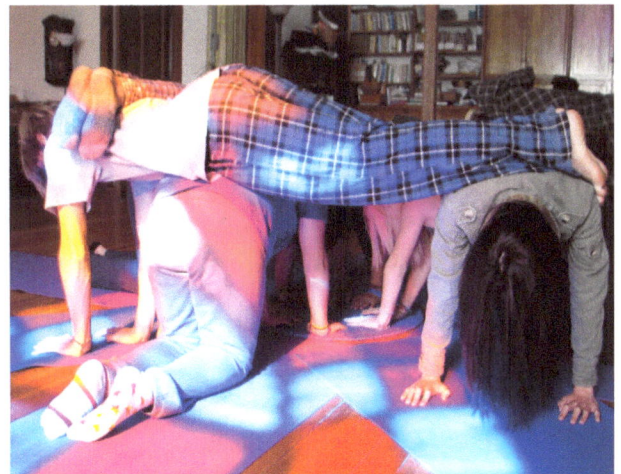

51

SUN WHEEL

This pose requires eight people, divided into two teams of four.

MOVEMENT INSTRUCTIONS:

* The bottom four people should be approximately the same size, height, and weight to create symmetry.

~These first four people (Team 1) stand in the four directions and face each other.

~Team 1 brings the hands and knees down until they are resting in Table Position.

~Team 1 should have their heads toward the center of the circle, close enough to almost touch.

* These tables become the support for Team 2

~ Team 2 stands on the left side of each table.

~ Members of Team 2 move down into Plank Pose with their feet resting on the low back of their "table partner."

~ The bottom team (the tables) support the top team (the planks).

* Plank Pose requires a good amount of upper body and core strength.

* Take care to exit the pose carefully and SLOWLY.

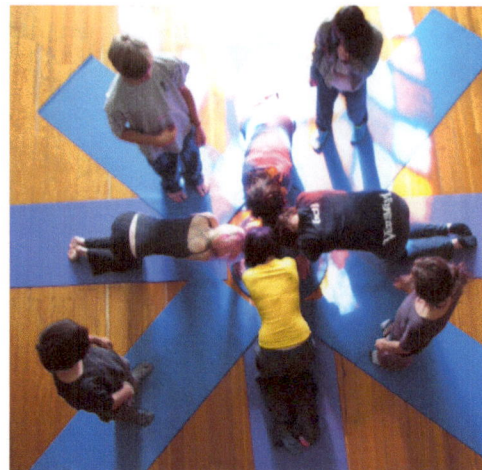

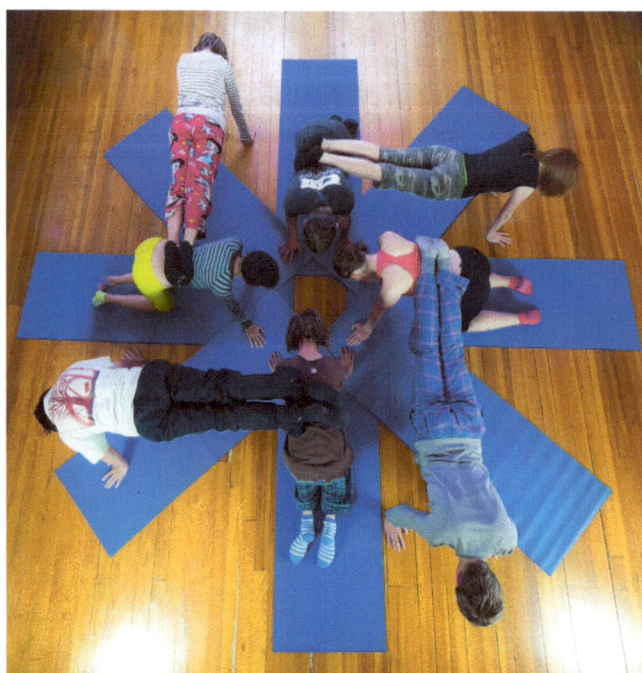

Frog Flower

This design requires five people.

Movement Instructions:

~ Begin with practitioners sitting in a circle on their knees. Open the knees slightly and bring the feet out from under the sitz bones.

~ Lower your torso back and down, carefully, toward the ground.

~ Connect the circle by holding both neighbors' hands.

> ** This is an intense posture. Do not attempt this pose if you have knee or lower back issues.*

> ** This is a deep stretch for the quadriceps and psoas muscles.*

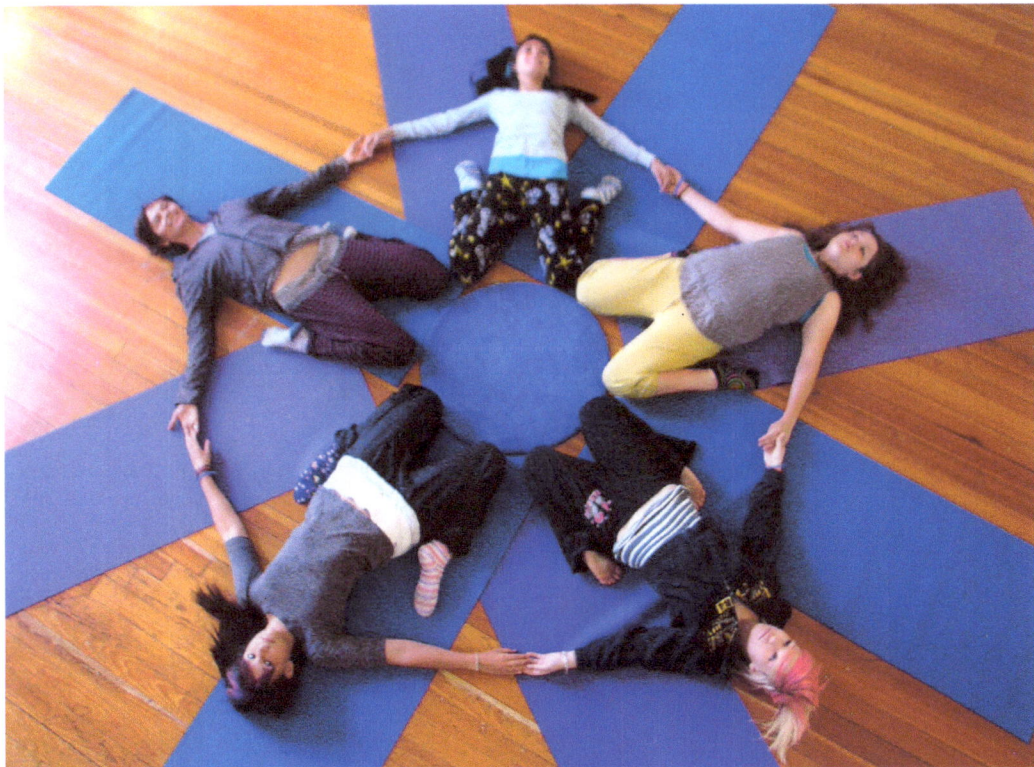

WATER BABIES

This pose requires eight people divided into two teams of four.

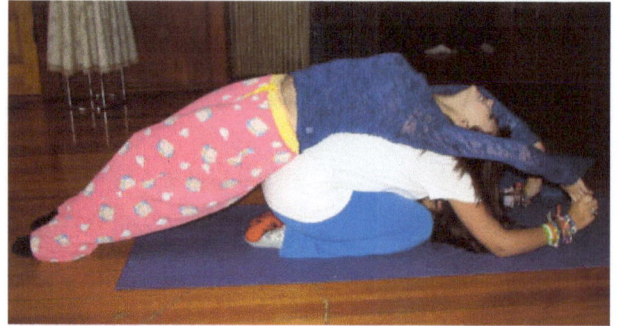

MOVEMENT INSTRUCTIONS:

~ Team 1: Begin in Child's Pose in each of the four directions, with the heads toward the center of the circle.

~ Team 2: Sit with the backs against each person in Team 1, facing out.

~ Next, participants from Team 2 rise to their feet with the knees bent, so that they can slowly move backwards to lie down over the pelvis and back of their Team 1 partner.

~ Team 2 straightens the legs and straightens the arms alongside the ears, stretching the arms toward the center of the circle.

> ** Straightening the legs creates more weight for the people in Team 1, so if the weight increase feels extreme, keep your legs bent. Make sure to communicate!*

~ The participants in the North/South position of Team 2 connect hands with each other. East/West does the same.

> ** This pose is a deep hip stretch for the support group (Team 1). Breathe deeply and sink your sitz bones down toward your heels.*

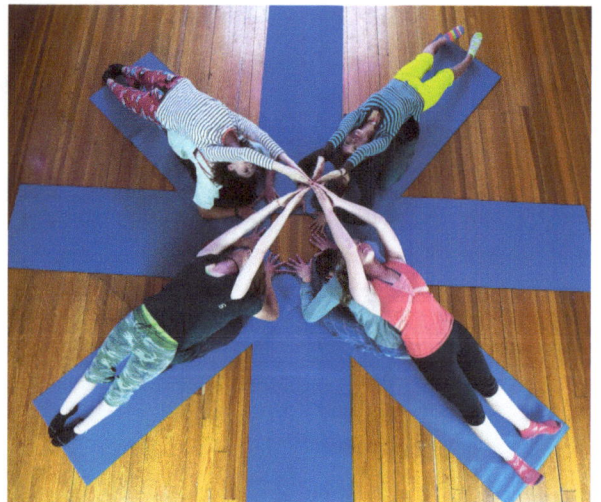

> ** This pose creates lengthening in the front of the body for members of Team 2. Take deep breaths, stretching and extending the limbs away from each other on the inhale.*

~ Exit this pose slowly. Team 1 may want to move the hips several times in a clockwise circular motion to integrate the stretch further into the hips. Then, switch the rotation of the hips.

> ** As always, when working with someone else it is very important to move slowly and maintain good communication to ensure that no one is going beyond his/her limit.*

> ** If the entire group consists of heavier/lighter people, participants should pair up with someone of relatively equal weight.*

~ Team 1 and 2 can change teams and repeat the actions of the pose.

Water strider: Variation on Water babies

This pose requires eight people.

Movement Instructions:

Begin in Water Babies.

~ From Water Babies, Team 2 (on top), bends the knees and places the feet on the ground.

> *Straightening the legs increases the front body stretch for team 2 but also increases the weight on Team 1. You may want to keep the knees bent and work up to straightening them.*

~ Next, participants in Team 2 connect hands with their neighbors and open the arms into a wide T.

> *This position creates a nice heart opening and a stretch for the chest.*

> *The arm placement (arms straight, hands joined) produces a square-shaped design.*

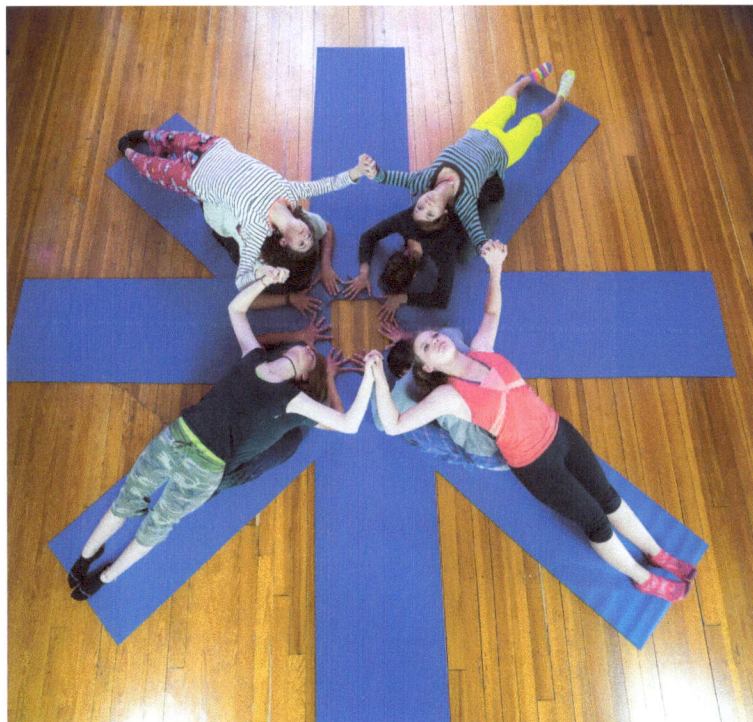

Variation
~All participants bend arms at right angles.

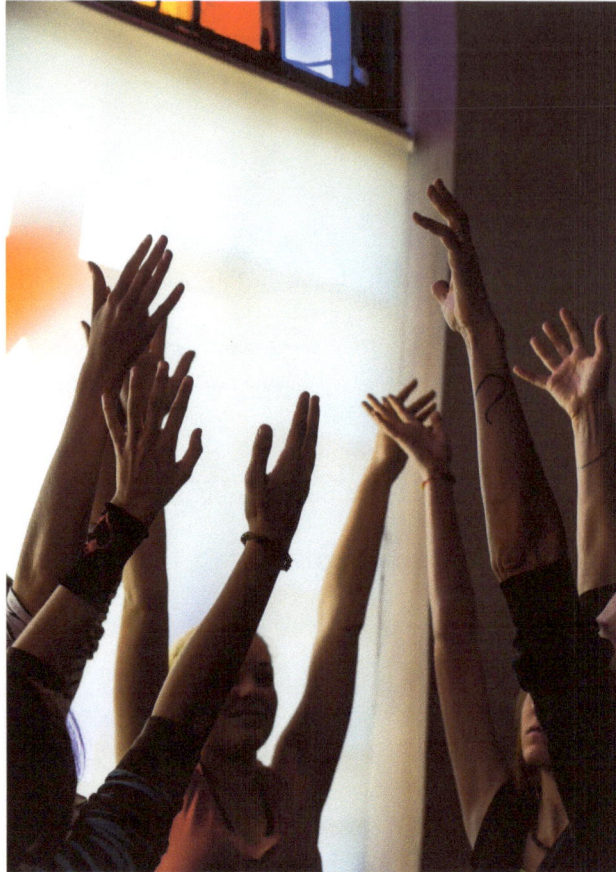

The story of Mandala Yoga begins as seed planted in soil; that, given love, water, and sun, grows to become a beautiful flower, a mandala.

My name is Juniper Bowers. I am a secondary Spanish language teacher and a certified yoga instructor. I teach both Spanish and yoga as electives at a small charter school in rural southwest New Mexico.

The mission of Aldo Leopold Charter High School, is to provide outdoor experience and inquiry-based education. Much of my job as a teacher is to ask meaningful questions, with the purpose of making the students think and to encourage them to ask questions that will ultimately lead the group to an appropriate answer.

So this story began, with the question I posed to my high school yoga class. I had practiced partner yoga over the years and loved the communicative aspects of two people working toward a common goal and I had wondered what yoga would be like with more than two people. How could one create a group dynamic focused around a common goal? I asked the class "What would it be like to practice yoga, not from an individual standpoint, but as a group? What would it look like, what would the experience feel like?"

There was talk around the circle of how to create poses using synchronized movement to strengthen the mind and body connection of the group and, because we use an outdoor education-based curriculum, we decided that we would create the pose designs based on forms in nature, or sacred geometry, and mandalas.

Once we decided on the goal, we needed to find a starting point. The class came up with the idea that the designs would begin with the four cardinal directions, which was logical for students that spend much of the year learning how to navigate in the wilderness. We placed four people in the positions of North, South, East and West. From here, the midpoints were discovered as a necessity since no persons arm span is long enough to reach the distance from West to North or from East to South. To create connection we needed the SE, SW, NE, and NW points: With these midpoints, the group could join hands. We connected, formed a circle and, like a globe with our points of reference, we opened up a whole new world of yoga. Finally, we had a template to begin our designs.

An inquiry into the nature of a mandala was our starting point. A simple definition of a mandala is a circumference that includes a perceived center, and it is from this center, that the circle opens outwardly and symmetrically. We brainstormed natural and man-made objects that opened up from a center point. As the list grew so did our appreciation for the world around us, "There are mandalas everywhere!" one student exclaimed. Another student said, "I am a mandala!" and continued with an explanation about how, from the navel, the human body is like a star. "Oh a star! A star is a mandala!" And on the students went, listing and exclaiming and learning and creating, giving shape to this book that blossomed like a lotus.

From our exploration of mandalas we began to look at examples of sacred geometry: shapes, squares, circles, triangles, stars, hexagrams, along with the combinations of circles within squares, triangles within hexagrams. These designs are called yantras. Part of the exploration of yantras was learning first to draw them on paper, using compasses and rulers and then emulating designs with our arms and legs as the lines to create the designs. Each inquiry naturally led to more questions and answers about the relationship between numbers and shapes.

We began to look at designs created by other cultures such as Native American, Egyptian, Aztec, Celtic and Viking. All of these cultures created mandalas, and some of the designs inspired a few of our poses and increased our awareness of different cultures and even geography. I could have never imagined the amount of interdisciplinary learning that would grow from that initial planted seed. We were practicing inquiry-based learning at its finest! I knew that I was watching something special and unique evolve, so I began to document the poses as they were created. I took pictures and recorded details and instructions on how to get into the poses.

This book is the product of five years of trial and error, fun and problem solving, inspiration and collaboration during which mandala yoga became the most popular elective class in the school. Mandala Yoga is an instruction manual, and it is written for anyone who has a group of people willing to come together to explore the idea of mandalas through movement.

The foundation poses of a mandala design are based on traditional yoga poses. Mountain, table, staff, and corpse pose begin each design and are a great way to focus one's awareness into the body before beginning the movement. Once the group grounds together, the movement begins, using the breath as a way to coordinate. Movement is very much like synchronized swimming on land. As the design emerges one can literally feel the beauty of the shape, and through stretching, strengthening and balancing, these poses bring a sense of calm focus to the mind and an opening of the heart. The poses themselves are designed with integrity and balance in mind. Once achieved, mandala poses are easy to sustain by the support and placement of the foundation. Each person creates a sense of balance through his or her presence. Working together to create balance requires teamwork, communication and problem solving skills. There are many factors to be taken into account to achieve each pose. Each person in the circle is a different height and weight, and may have differing levels of ability, strength, or flexibility. All of these factors are balanced out by each person's placement in the circle. Proper alignment of the hands and feet and the ability to find a center of gravity, as well as group awareness and accommodation, are essential to the pose's success. Much like the movements of partner yoga, deeper stretches can be attained by the shared weight. Mandala Yoga is a process. It is playful and breaks down physical and even emotional barriers by providing a safe, open platform to give and receive touch. The bonds that are formed within a mandala circle are deep because it is an unusual and meaningful experience for all participants. Whether you practice mandala yoga once, or weekly, it is an experience that stays with you and changes you. The students, by the end of the semester, gained in self-confidence and body awareness, and they bonded deeply with each other. They left the class with a spring in their step, and many, even after graduating, still practice yoga on their own.

During my experience teaching this class, I have watched a new group of students bond, laugh, learn and stretch together each new semester. I began to be curious what it would be like to do mandala yoga with other people in my community. I thought they might benefit in the same way as my students. Do others need a positive platform for connection as well? So I began a community mandala class in a park downtown. I placed fliers around town and waited to see what kind of response I would get. Each week, a few people trickled in, curious about what mandala yoga was about. I would hear comments like, "That was fun!" Or, "What a nice way to meet people," and, " How cool to feel connection with strangers!" One participant told me, "I could feel my boundary issues melting away." Overall I learned that participants felt energized by the whole group, and had never experienced anything like it!

These sentiments and the expressions of gratitude from the people who participated in mandala yoga verified what I already knew: We all need a way to play, to be active, to be social, and to give and receive physical contact. The world that we live in is increasingly sedentary, socially awkward, and isolating. Social media is not the same as true face to face connection, multi-player video games are not truly playful, and sitting in front of a screen is not good for overall well-being. We need to incorporate and encourage ways and means to feel real connection with each other to foster a sense of humanity, to care about what happens to our environment and to create a better world. The mandala becomes much more than just a fun activity. Rather, it becomes a metaphor for embarking on a journey into the unknown by means of the known: human contact and sacred geometry. Much like the seed of life design, it continues to grow, circles upon circles, and gives birth to the flower of life, or infinite possibility. Mandala yoga can connect us all with this science and with this magic.

Whether you are a teacher or a yogi does not matter, what matters is that the mandala speaks to you. There are as many ways to apply these poses as there are people who use them. Get creative! I have used mandala yoga as a summer camp activity, as a team and community builder, as an after school program, with home school groups, and at festivals to draw people together. I invite you to get inspired by this story and these poses, find a group of people to practice with, and create even more designs. Just let the mandala move you, and see what may flower...

With Gratitude,
Juniper Bowers

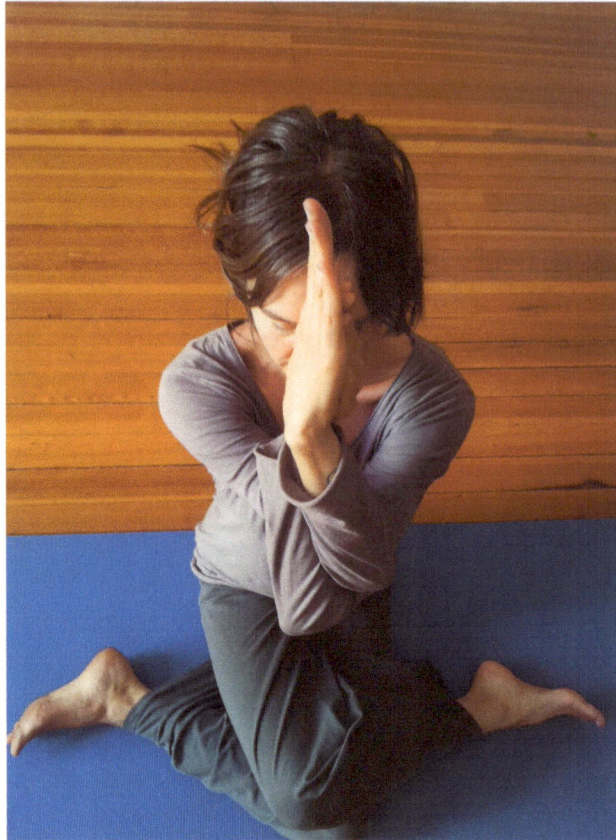

About the Author

Juniper Bowers is a certified yoga instructor and a licensed secondary educator who has been teaching for over 20 years.

She began her career in education as a high school Spanish teacher. When Juniper received her Yoga training at Inner Gate Yoga, she was drawn immediately to teaching yoga to children. Her first yoga curriculum for kids, InterActive Anatomy, combines the study of anatomy through movement. Juniper began teaching InterActive Anatomy as a summer program class and eventually began teaching the class at Aldo Leopold Charter High School in Silver City, NM as an elective.

The class evolved to become Mandala Yoga, which includes group yoga and team building exercises, along with the study of mandalas, art, sacred geometry, and even rhythmic clapping games and "brain gym." This book is a compilation of the poses created by the class.

Juniper lives in Mimbres, New Mexico, with her husband Daniel and her two kids, Escher and Semilla. She loves to practice Yoga and Thai massage/Rossiter and has written three yoga curriculums for children: InterActive Anatomy, Mandala Yoga, and Alphabet in Action.

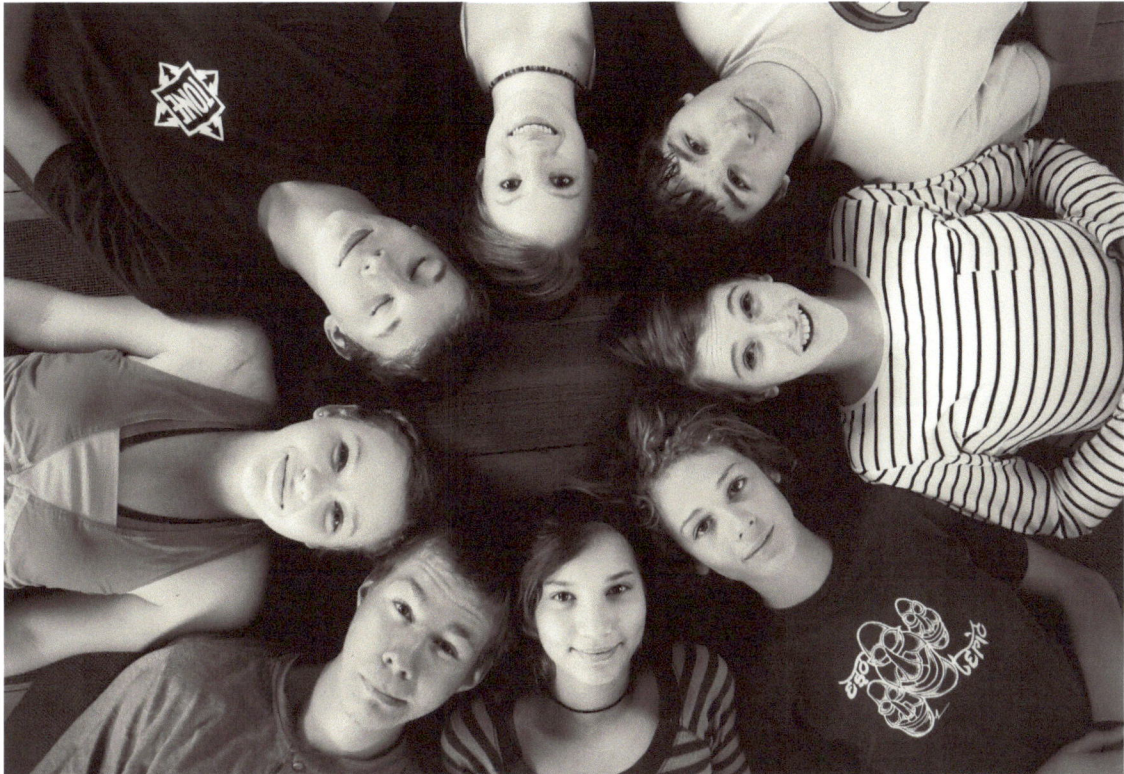

Special thanks to Aldo Leopold High School in Silver City, New Mexico

© 2016 Juniper Bowers

Written by Juniper Bowers
Photos taken by Daniel Freeman, Escher Bowers, Jay Hempell, Josh Stretch
Illustrations by Elli Sorenson
Page Layout Design and Cover Design by Isaac Clodfelter
Edited by Antoinette Durham of Durham Editors

For more information about Mandala Yoga Curriculum:
Send an e-mail to *dandjune@yahoo.com*
Subscribe to our Youtube channel — **"Juniper Bowers"**
Visit us at MANDALAKIDS.COM

www.ingramcontent.com/pod-product-compliance
Lightning Source LLC
Chambersburg PA
CBHW060807270326
41927CB00003B/85